ACLS
Advanced Cardiac Life Support
Provider Handbook

By Dr. Karl Dis-
que

Presented by the:

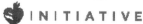
Save a Life
INITIATIVE

Educational Service Disclaimer

This Provider Handbook is an educational service provided by Satori Continuum Publishing. Use of this service is governed by the terms and conditions provided below. Please read the statements below carefully before accessing or using the service. By accessing or using this service, you agree to be bound by all of the terms and conditions herein.

The material contained in this Provider Handbook does not contain standards that are intended to be applied rigidly and explicitly followed in all cases. A health care professional's judgment must remain central to the selection of diagnostic tests and therapy options of a specific patient's medical condition. Ultimately, all liability associated with the utilization of any of the information presented here rests solely and completely with the health care provider utilizing the service.

Version 2020.01

TABLE *of* CONTENTS

Chapter 1 Introduction to ACLS **5**

2 The Initial Assessment **6**

3 Basic Life Support **7**

Initiating the Chain of Survival – 7
2015 BLS Guideline Changes – 8
2010 BLS Guideline Changes – 9
BLS for Adults – 10
One-Rescuer Adult BLS/CPR
Two-Rescuer Adult BLS/CPR
Adult Mouth-to-Mask Ventilation
Adult Bag-Mask Ventilation in Two-Rescuer CPR
Self-Assessment for BLS – 16

4 Advanced Cardiac Life Support **18**

Normal Heart Anatomy and Physiology – 18
The ACLS Survey (ABCD) – 19
Airway Management – 20
Basic Airway Adjuncts
Basic Airway Technique
Advanced Airway Adjuncts
Routes of Access – 24
Intravenous Route
Intraosseous Route
Pharmacological Tools – 25
Self-Assessment for ACLS – 26

5 Principles of Early Defibrillation **27**

Keys to Using an Automated External Defibrillator – 28
Criteria to Apply AED
Basic AED Operation

6 Systems of Care **30**

Cardiopulmonary Resuscitation – 31
Initiating the Chain of Survival
Post-Cardiac Arrest Care – 32
Therapeutic Hypothermia
Optimization of Hemodynamics and Ventilation
Percutaneous Coronary Intervention
Neurologic Care
Acute Coronary Syndrome – 33
Goals of ACS Treatment
Acute Stroke – 34
Goals of Acute Ischemic Stroke Care
The Resuscitation Team – 35
Education, Implementation, Teams – 36
Self-Assessment for Systems of Care – 37

TABLE *of* CONTENTS

Chapter **7** ACLS Cases **38**

Respiratory Arrest – 38
Ventricular Fibrillation and Pulseless Ventricular Tachycardia – 42
Pulseless Electrical Activity and Asystole – 44
Post-Cardiac Arrest Care – 48
  Blood Pressure Support and Vasopressors
  Hypothermia
Symptomatic Bradycardia – 51
Tachycardia – 54
  Symptomatic Tachycardia with Heart Rate Greater than 100 BPM
  Stable and Unstable Tachycardia
Acute Coronary Syndrome – 58
Acute Stroke – 60
Self-Assessment for ACLS Cases – 64

8 ACLS Essentials **67**

9 Additional Tools **68**

MediCode – 68
CertAlert+ – 68

10 ACLS Review Questions **69**

INTRODUCTION TO ACLS

The goal of Advanced Cardiovascular Life Support (ACLS) is to achieve the best possible outcome for individuals who are experiencing a life-threatening event. ACLS is a series of evidence-based responses simple enough to be committed to memory and recalled under moments of stress. These ACLS protocols have been developed through research, patient case studies, clinical studies, and opinions of experts in the field. The gold standard in the United States and other countries is the course curriculum published by the American Heart Association (AHA).

Previously, the AHA released periodic updates to their Cardiopulmonary Resuscitation (CPR) and Emergency Cardiovascular Care (ECC) guidelines on a five-year cycle, with the most recent update published in 2015. Moving forward, the AHA will no longer wait five years between updates; instead, it will maintain the most up-to-date recommendations online at ECCguidelines.heart.org. Health care providers are recommended to supplement the materials presented in this handbook with the guidelines published by the AHA and refer to the most current interventions and rationales throughout their study of ACLS.

 Take Note

Refer to the Basic Life Support (BLS) Provider Handbook, also presented by the Save a Life Initiative, for a more comprehensive review of the BLS Survey. This handbook specifically covers ACLS algorithms and only briefly describes BLS. All ACLS providers are presumed capable of performing BLS correctly. While this handbook covers BLS basics, it is essential that ACLS providers be proficient in BLS first.

While ACLS providers should always be mindful of timeliness, it is important to provide the intervention that most appropriately fits the needs of the individual. Proper utilization of ACLS requires rapid and accurate assessment of the individual's condition. This not only applies to the provider's initial assessment of an individual in distress, but also to the reassessment throughout the course of treatment with ACLS.

ACLS protocols assume that the provider may not have all of the information needed from the individual or all of the resources needed to properly use ACLS in all cases. For example, if a provider is utilizing ACLS on the side of the road, they will not have access to sophisticated devices to measure breathing or arterial blood pressure. Nevertheless, in such situations, ACLS providers have the framework to provide the best possible care in the given circumstances. ACLS algorithms are based on past performances and result in similar life-threatening cases and are intended to achieve the best possible outcome for the individual during emergencies. The foundation of all algorithms involves the systematic approach of the BLS Survey and the ACLS Survey (using steps ABCD) that you will find later in this handbook.

>> *Next: The Initial Assessment*

THE INITIAL ASSESSMENT

Determining whether an individual is conscious or unconscious can be done very quickly. If you notice someone in distress, lying down in a public place, or possibly injured, call out to them.

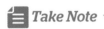 **Take Note**

- Make sure the scene is safe before approaching the individual and conducting the BLS or ACLS Survey.

- When encountering an individual who is "down," the first assessment to make is whether they are conscious or unconscious.

If the individual is unconscious, then start with the BLS Survey and move on to the ACLS Survey. If they are conscious, then start with the ACLS Survey.

>> *Next: Basic Life Support*

BASIC LIFE SUPPORT

The AHA has updated the Basic Life Support (BLS) course over the years as new research in cardiac care has become available. Cardiac arrest continues to be a leading cause of death in the United States. BLS guidelines have changed dramatically, and the elements of BLS continue to be some of the most important steps in initial treatment. General concepts of BLS include:

- Quickly starting the Chain of Survival.
- Delivering high-quality chest compressions for adults, children, and infants.
- Knowing where to locate and understanding how to use an Automatic External Defibrillator (AED)
- Providing rescue breathing when appropriate.
- Understanding how to perform as a team.
- Knowing how to treat choking.

INITIATING THE CHAIN OF SURVIVAL

Early initiation of BLS has been shown to increase the probability of survival for an individual dealing with cardiac arrest. To increase the odds of surviving a cardiac event, the rescuer should follow the steps in the Adult Chain of Survival *(Figure 1)*.

Adult Chain of Survival

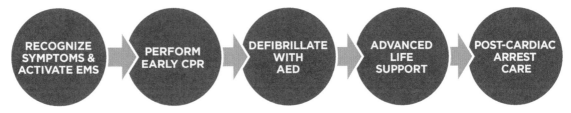

Figure 1

>> Next: Pediatric Chain of Survival

Emergencies in children and infants are not usually caused by the heart. Children and infants most often have breathing problems that trigger cardiac arrest. The first and most important step of the Pediatric Chain of Survival *(Figure 2)* is prevention.

Pediatric Chain of Survival

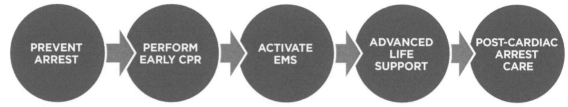

Figure 2

2015 BLS GUIDELINE CHANGES

In 2015, the AHA update to its Emergency Cardiovascular Care (ECC) guidelines strengthened some of the recommendations made in 2010. For an in-depth review of the changes made, refer to the AHA's executive summary document.

Below are the details of the changes made to 2015 guidelines for BLS:

- The change from the traditional ABC (Airway, Breathing, Compressions) sequence in 2010 to the CAB (Compressions, Airway, Breathing) sequence was confirmed in the 2015 guidelines. The emphasis on early initiation of chest compressions without delay for airway assessment or rescue breathing has resulted in improved outcomes.

- Previously, rescuers may have been faced with the choice of leaving the individual to activate emergency medical services (EMS). Now, rescuers are likely to have a cellular phone, often with speakerphone capabilities. The use of a speakerphone or other hands-free device allows the rescuer to continue rendering aid while communicating with the EMS dispatcher.

- Untrained rescuers should initiate hands-only CPR under the direction of the EMS dispatcher as soon as the individual is identified as unresponsive.

- Trained rescuers should continue to provide CPR with rescue breathing.

- In situations where unresponsiveness is thought to be from narcotic overdose, trained BLS rescuers may administer naloxone via the intranasal or intramuscular route, if the drug is available. For individuals without a pulse, this should be done after CPR is initiated.

- The importance of high-quality chest compressions was confirmed, with enhanced recommendations for maximum rates and depths.

    - Chest compressions should be delivered at a rate of 100 to 120 per minute because compressions faster than 120 per minute may not allow for cardiac refill and reduce perfusion.

    - Chest compressions should be delivered to adults at a depth between 2 to 2.4 inches (5 to 6 cm) because compressions at greater depths may result in injury to vital organs without increasing odds of survival.

    - Chest compressions should be delivered to children (less than one-year-old) at a depth of one third the chest, usually about 1.5 to 2 inches (4 to 5 cm).

    - Rescuers must allow for full chest recoil in between compressions to promote cardiac filling.

>> Next: 2015 BLS Guideline Changes Continued

- Because it is difficult to accurately judge quality of chest compressions, an audiovisual feedback device may be used to optimize delivery of CPR during resuscitation.
    - Interruptions of chest compressions, including pre- and post-AED shocks, should be as short as possible.
- Compression to ventilation ratio remains 30:2 for an individual without an advanced airway in place.
- Individuals with an advanced airway in place should receive uninterrupted chest compressions with ventilation being delivered at a rate of one every six seconds.
- In cardiac arrest, the defibrillator should be used as soon as possible.
- Chest compressions should be resumed as soon as a shock is delivered.
- Biphasic defibrillators are more effective in terminating life-threatening rhythms and are preferred to older monophasic defibrillators.
- Energy settings vary by manufacturer, and the device specific guidelines should be followed.
- Standard dose epinephrine (1 mg every 3 to 5 min) is the preferred vasopressor. High dose epinephrine and vasopressin have not been shown to be more effective, and therefore, are not recommended.
- For cardiac arrest that is suspected to be caused by coronary artery blockage, angiography should be performed emergently.
- Targeted temperature management should maintain a constant temperature between 32 to 36 degrees C for at least 24 hours in the hospital environment.
- Routine cooling of individuals in the prehospital environment is not recommended.

2010 BLS GUIDELINE CHANGES

These following represent a summary of the 2010 changes:

- Previously, the initial steps were Airway, Breathing, Compressions, or ABC. The literature indicates that starting compressions early in the process will increase survival rates. Therefore, the steps have been changed to Compressions, Airway, Breathing, or CAB. This is intended to encourage early CPR and avoid bystanders interpreting agonal breathing as signs of life and withholding CPR.
- "Look, listen, and feel" for breathing is no longer recommended. Instead of assessing the person's breathing, begin CPR if the person is not breathing (or is only gasping for breath), has no pulse (or if you are unsure), or is unresponsive. Do not perform an initial assessment of respirations. The goal is early delivery of chest compressions to cardiac arrest persons.
- High-quality CPR consists of the following:
    - Keep compression rate of 100 to 120 beats per minute for all persons.
    - Keep compression depth between 2 to 2.4 inches for adults and children, and about 1.5 inches for infants.
    - Allow complete chest recoil after each compression.
    - Minimize interruptions in CPR, except to use an AED or to change rescuer positions.
    - Do not over ventilate.
    - Provide CPR as a team when possible.

>> Next: 2010 BLS Guideline Changes Continued

- Cricoid pressure is no longer routinely performed.
- Pulse checks are shorter. Feel for a pulse for no more than 10 seconds; if a pulse is absent or if you are not sure you feel a pulse, then begin compressions. Even trained clinicians cannot always reliably tell if they can feel a pulse.
- For infants, use a manual defibrillator if available. If not available, an AED with pediatric dose attenuator should be used for an infant. If an AED with dose attenuator is not available, then use an adult AED, even for an infant.

BLS FOR ADULTS

BLS for adults focuses on doing several tasks simultaneously. In previous versions of BLS, the focus was primarily on one-rescuer CPR. In many situations, more than one person is available to do CPR. This simultaneous and choreographed method includes performing chest compressions, managing the airway, delivering rescue breaths, and using the AED, all as a team. By coordinating efforts, a team of rescuers can save valuable seconds when time lost equals damage to the heart and brain.

Simple Adult BLS Algorithm

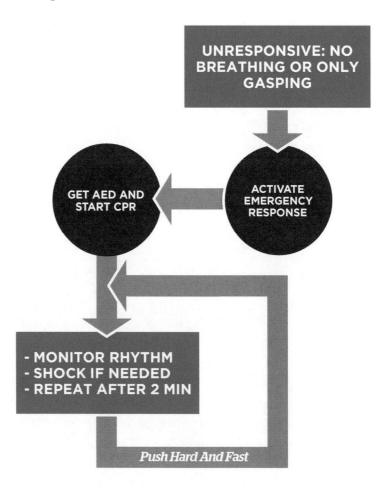

Figure 3

>> Next: One-Rescuer BLS/CPR for Adults

ONE-RESCUER BLS/CPR FOR ADULTS

Be Safe

- Move the person out of traffic.
- Move the person out of water and dry the person. (Drowning persons should be removed from the water and dried off; they should also be removed from standing water, such as puddles, pools, gutters, etc.)
- Be sure you do not become injured yourself.

Assess the Person

- Shake the person and talk to them loudly.
- Check to see if the person is breathing. (Agonal breathing, which is occasional gasping and is ineffective, does not count as breathing.)

Call EMS

- Send someone for help and to get an AED.
- If alone, call for help while assessing for breathing and pulse. (The AHA emphasizes that cell phones are available everywhere now and most have a built-in speakerphone. Call for help without leaving the person.)

CPR

- Check pulse.
- Begin chest compressions and delivering breaths.

Defibrillate

- Attach the AED when available.
- Listen and perform the steps as directed.

>> Next: CPR STEPS

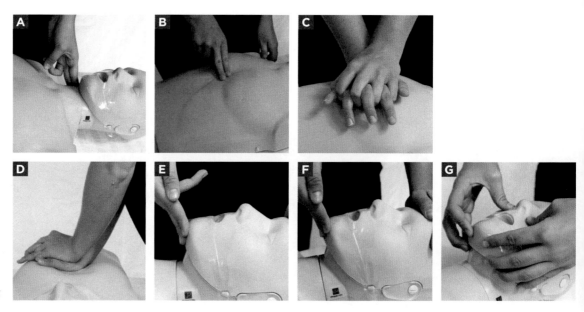

Figure 4

CPR Steps

1. Check for the carotid pulse on the side of the neck. Keep in mind not to waste time trying to feel for a pulse; feel for no more than 10 seconds. If you are not sure you feel a pulse, begin CPR with a cycle of 30 chest compressions and two breaths *(Figure 4a)*.

2. Use the heel of one hand on the lower half of the sternum in the middle of the chest *(Figure 4b)*.

3. Put your other hand on top of the first hand *(Figure 4c)*.

4. Straighten your arms and press straight down *(Figure 4d)*. Compressions should be at least two inches into the person's chest and at a rate of 100 to 120 compressions per minute.

5. Be sure that between each compression you completely stop pressing on the chest and allow the chest wall to return to its natural position. Leaning or resting on the chest between compressions can keep the heart from refilling in between each compression and make CPR less effective.

6. After 30 compressions, stop compressions and open the airway by tilting the head and lifting the chin *(Figure 4e & 4f)*.

    a. Put your hand on the person's forehead and tilt the head back.

    b. Lift the person's jaw by placing your index and middle fingers on the lower jaw; lift up.

    c. Do not perform the head-tilt/chin-lift maneuver if you suspect the person may have a neck injury. In that case, the jaw-thrust is used.

    d. For the jaw-thrust maneuver, grasp the angles of the lower jaw and lift it with both hands, one on each side, moving the jaw forward. If their lips are closed, open the lower lip using your thumb *(Figure 4g)*.

7. Give a breath while watching the chest rise. Repeat while giving a second breath. Breaths should be delivered over one second.

8. Resume chest compressions. Switch quickly between compressions and rescue breaths to minimize interruptions in chest compressions.

>> Next: Two-Rescuer BLS/CPR for Adults

TWO-RESCUER BLS/CPR FOR ADULTS

Many times there will be a second person available who can act as a rescuer. The AHA emphasizes that cell phones are available everywhere now and most have a built-in speakerphone. Direct the second rescuer to call 911 without leaving the person while you begin CPR. This second rescuer can also find an AED while you stay with the person. When the second rescuer returns, the CPR tasks can be shared:

1. The second rescuer prepares the AED for use.

2. You begin chest compressions and count the compressions out loud.

3. The second rescuer applies the AED pads.

4. The second rescuer opens the person's airway and gives rescue breaths.

5. Switch roles after every five cycles of compressions and breaths. One cycle consists of 30 compressions and two breaths.

6. Be sure that between each compression you completely stop pressing on the chest and allow the chest wall to return to its natural position. Leaning or resting on the chest between compressions can keep the heart from refilling in between each compression and make CPR less effective. Rescuers who become tired may tend to lean on the chest more during compressions; switching roles helps rescuers perform high-quality compressions.

7. Quickly switch between roles to minimize interruptions in delivering chest compressions.

8. When the AED is connected, minimize interruptions of CPR by switching rescuers while the AED analyzes the heart rhythm. If a shock is indicated, minimize interruptions in CPR. Resume CPR as soon as possible.

>> Next: Adult Mouth-to-Mask Ventilation

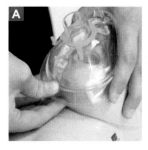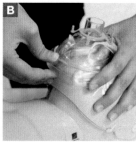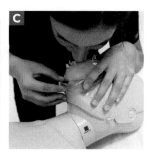

Figure 5

ADULT MOUTH-TO-MASK VENTILATION

In one-rescuer CPR, breaths should be supplied using a pocket mask, if available.

1. Give 30 high-quality chest compressions.

2. Seal the mask against the person's face by placing four fingers of one hand across the top of the mask and the thumb of the other hand along the bottom edge of the mask *(Figure 5a)*.

3. Using the fingers of your hand on the bottom of the mask, open the airway using the head-tilt/chin-lift maneuver. (Do not do this if you suspect the person may have a neck injury) *(Figure 5b)*.

4. Press firmly around the edges of the mask and ventilate by delivering a breath over one second as you watch the person's chest rise *(Figure 5c)*.

5. Practice using the bag valve mask; it is essential to forming a tight seal and delivering

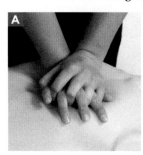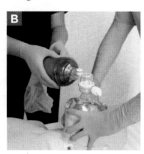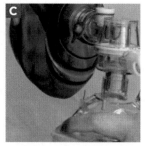

Figure 6

ADULT BAG-MASK VENTILATION IN TWO-RESCUER CPR

If two people are present and a bag-mask device is available, the second rescuer is positioned at the victim's head while the other rescuer performs high-quality chest compressions. Give 30 high-quality chest compressions.

1. Deliver 30 high-quality chest compressions while counting out loud *(Figure 6a)*.

2. The second rescuer holds the bag-mask with one hand using the thumb and index finger in the shape of a "C" on one side of the mask to form a seal between the mask and the face, while the other fingers open the airway by lifting the person's lower jaw *(Figure 6b)*.

3. The second rescuer gives two breaths over one second each *(Figure 6c)*.

>> Next: Simple Adult BLS Algorithm

Simple Adult BLS Algorithm

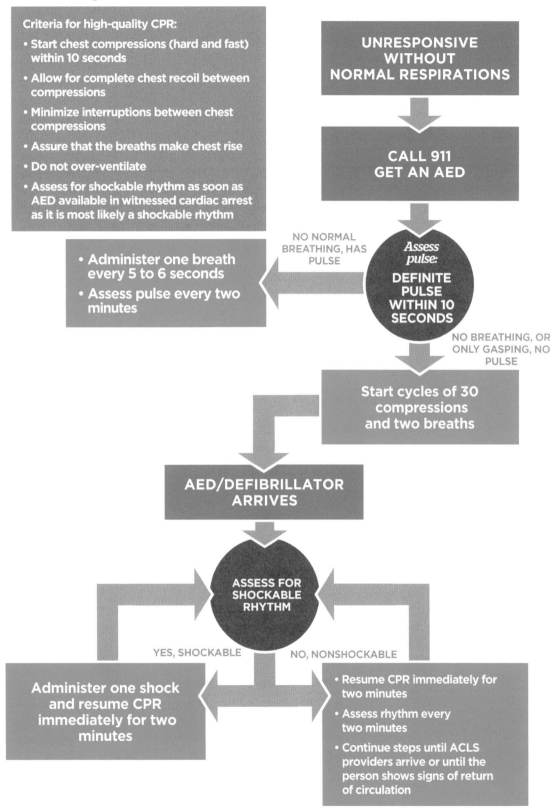

Criteria for high-quality CPR:

- Start chest compressions (hard and fast) within 10 seconds
- Allow for complete chest recoil between compressions
- Minimize interruptions between chest compressions
- Assure that the breaths make chest rise
- Do not over-ventilate
- Assess for shockable rhythm as soon as AED available in witnessed cardiac arrest as it is most likely a shockable rhythm

UNRESPONSIVE WITHOUT NORMAL RESPIRATIONS

CALL 911 GET AN AED

Assess pulse: **DEFINITE PULSE WITHIN 10 SECONDS**

NO NORMAL BREATHING, HAS PULSE

- Administer one breath every 5 to 6 seconds
- Assess pulse every two minutes

NO BREATHING, OR ONLY GASPING, NO PULSE

Start cycles of 30 compressions and two breaths

AED/DEFIBRILLATOR ARRIVES

ASSESS FOR SHOCKABLE RHYTHM

YES, SHOCKABLE

NO, NONSHOCKABLE

Administer one shock and resume CPR immediately for two minutes

- Resume CPR immediately for two minutes
- Assess rhythm every two minutes
- Continue steps until ACLS providers arrive or until the person shows signs of return of circulation

Figure 7

>> *Next: Self-Assessment for BLS*

1. Which of the following is true regarding BLS?
   a. It is obsolete.
   b. Recent changes prohibit mouth-to-mouth.
   c. It should be mastered prior to ACLS.
   d. It has little impact on survival.

2. What is the first step in the assessment of an individual found "down"?
   a. Check their blood pressure.
   b. Check their heart rate.
   c. Check to see if they are conscious or unconscious.
   d. Check their pupil size.

3. What factor is critical in any emergency situation?
   a. Scene safety
   b. Age of the individual
   c. Resuscitation status
   d. Pregnancy status

4. How did the BLS guidelines change with the recent AHA update?
   a. Ventilations are performed before compressions.
   b. ABC is now CAB.
   c. Use of an AED is no longer recommended.
   d. Rapid transport is recommended over on-scene CPR.

5. Arrange the BLS Chain of Survival in the proper order:
   a. Look, listen, and feel
   b. Check responsiveness, call EMS and get AED, defibrillation, and circulation
   c. Check responsiveness, call EMS and get AED, chest compressions, and early defibrillation
   d. Call for help, shock, check pulse, shock, and transport

6. After activating EMS and sending someone for an AED, which of the following is correct for one-rescuer BLS of an unresponsive individual with no pulse?
   a. Start rescue breathing.
   b. Apply AED pads.
   c. Run to get help.
   d. Begin chest compressions.

ANSWERS

1. C

   ACLS providers are presumed to have mastered BLS skills. CPR is a critical part of resuscitating cardiac arrest victims.

2. C

   When responding to an individual who is "down," first determine if they are conscious or not. That determination dictates whether you start the BLS Survey or the ACLS Survey.

3. A

   Always assess the safety of the scene in any emergency situation. Do not become injured yourself.

4. B

   The focus is on early intervention and starting CPR. Look, listen, and feel has been removed to encourage performance of chest compressions.

5. C

   The focus is on early CPR and defibrillation.

6. D

   An unresponsive adult without a pulse must receive CPR, and chest compressions should be initiated immediately followed by ventilation.

>> Next: Advanced Cardiac Life Support

4 ADVANCED CARDIAC LIFE SUPPORT

NORMAL HEART ANATOMY AND PHYSIOLOGY

Understanding normal cardiac anatomy and physiology is an important component of performing ACLS. The heart is a hollow muscle comprised of four chambers surrounded by thick walls of tissue (septum). The atria are the two upper chambers and the ventricles are the two lower chambers. The left and right halves of the heart work together to pump blood throughout the body. The right atrium (RA) and the right ventricle (RV) pump deoxygenated blood to the lungs where it becomes oxygenated. This oxygen-rich blood returns to the left atrium (LA) and then enters the left ventricle (LV). The LV is the main pump that delivers the newly oxygenated blood to the rest of the body. Blood leaves the heart through a large vessel known as the aorta. Valves between each pair of connected chambers prevent the backflow of blood. The two atria contract simultaneously, as do the ventricles, making the contractions of the heart go from top to bottom. Each beat

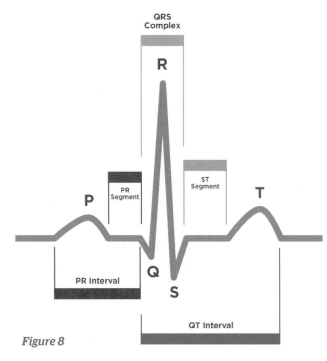

Figure 8

begins in the RA. The LV is the largest and thickest-walled of the four chambers, as it is responsible for pumping the newly oxygenated blood to the rest of the body. The sinoatrial (SA) node in the RA creates the electrical activity that acts as the heart's natural pacemaker. This electrical impulse then travels to the atrioventricular (AV) node, which lies between the atria and ventricles. After pausing there briefly, the electrical impulse moves on to the His – Purkinje system, which acts like wiring to conduct the electrical signal into the LV and RV. This electrical signal causes the heart muscle to contract and pump blood.

By understanding the normal electrical function of the heart, it will be easy to understand abnormal functions. When blood enters the atria of the heart, an electrical impulse that is sent out from the SA node conducts through the atria resulting in atrial contraction.

>> Next: Normal Heart Anatomy and Physiology

This atrial contraction registers on an electrocardiogram (ECG) strip as the P wave. This impulse then travels to the AV node, which in turn conducts the electrical impulse through the Bundle of His, bundle branches, and Purkinje fibers of the ventricles causing ventricular contraction. The time between the start of atrial contraction and the start of ventricular contraction registers on an ECG strip as the PR interval. The ventricular contraction registers on the ECG strip as the QRS complex. Following ventricular contraction, the ventricles rest and repolarize, which is registered on the ECG strip as the T wave. The atria also repolarize, but this coincides with the QRS complex, and therefore, cannot be observed on the ECG strip. Together a P wave, QRS complex, and T wave at proper intervals are indicative of normal sinus rhythm (NSR) *(Figure 8)*. Abnormalities that are in the conduction system can cause delays in the transmission of the electrical impulse and are detected on the ECG. These deviations from normal conduction can result in dysrhythmias such as heart blocks, pauses, tachycardias and bradycardias, blocks, and dropped beats. These rhythm disturbances will be covered in more detail further in the handbook.

THE ACLS SURVEY (A-B-C-D)

AIRWAY

Monitor and maintain an open airway at all times. The provider must decide if the benefit of adding an advanced airway outweighs the risk of pausing CPR. If the individual's chest is rising without using an advanced airway, continue giving CPR without pausing. However, if you are in a hospital or near trained professionals who can efficiently insert and use the airway, consider pausing CPR.

BREATHING

In cardiac arrest, administer 100% oxygen. Keep blood O2 saturation (sats) greater than or equal to 94 percent as measured by a pulse oximeter. Use quantitative waveform capnography when possible. Normal partial pressure of CO_2 is between 35 to 40 mmHg. High-quality CPR should produce a CO2 between 10 to 20 mmHg. If the ETCO2 reading is less than 10 mmHg after 20 minutes of CPR for an intubated individual, then you may consider stopping resuscitation attempts.

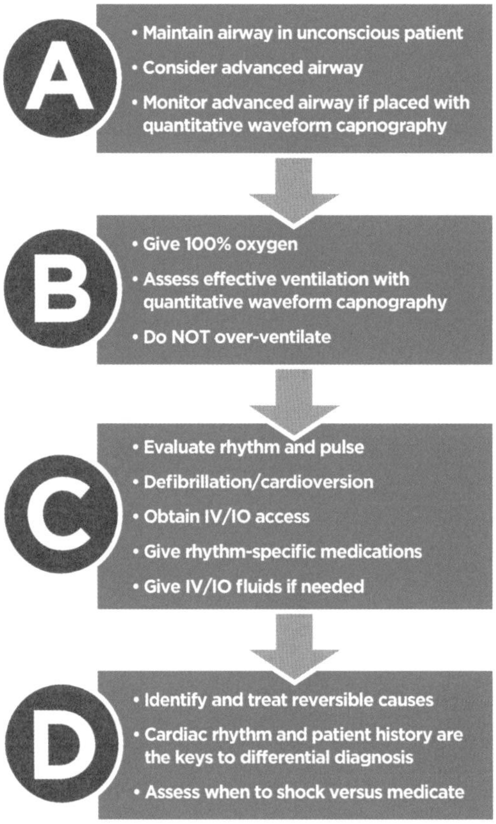

A
- Maintain airway in unconscious patient
- Consider advanced airway
- Monitor advanced airway if placed with quantitative waveform capnography

B
- Give 100% oxygen
- Assess effective ventilation with quantitative waveform capnography
- Do NOT over-ventilate

C
- Evaluate rhythm and pulse
- Defibrillation/cardioversion
- Obtain IV/IO access
- Give rhythm-specific medications
- Give IV/IO fluids if needed

D
- Identify and treat reversible causes
- Cardiac rhythm and patient history are the keys to differential diagnosis
- Assess when to shock versus medicate

Figure 9

CIRCULATION

Obtain intravenous (IV) access, when possible; intraosseous access (IO) is also acceptable. Monitor blood pressure with a blood pressure cuff or intra-arterial line if available. Monitor the heart rhythm using pads and a cardiac monitor. When using an AED, follow the directions (i.e., shock a shockable rhythm). Give fluids when appropriate. Use cardiovascular medications when indicated.

DIFFERENTIAL DIAGNOSIS

Start with the most likely cause of the arrest and then assess for less likely causes. Treat reversible causes and continue CPR as you create a differential diagnosis. Stop only briefly to confirm a diagnosis or to treat reversible causes. Minimizing interruptions in perfusion is key.

>> Next: Airway Management

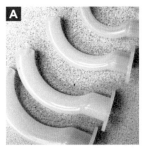 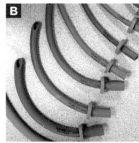 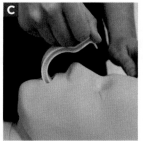 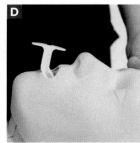

Figure 10

AIRWAY MANAGEMENT

If bag-mask ventilation is adequate, providers may defer insertion of an advanced airway. Health care providers should make the decision as to the appropriateness of placing an advanced airway during the ACLS Survey. The value of securing the airway must be balanced against the need to minimize the interruption in perfusion that results in halting CPR during airway placement.

Basic airway equipment includes the oropharyngeal airway (OPA) and the nasopharyngeal airway (NPA). The primary difference between an OPA *(Figure 10a)* and an NPA *(Figure 10b)* is that an OPA is placed in the mouth *(Figure 11c and 11d)* while an NPA is inserted through the nose. Both airway equipment terminate in the pharynx. The main advantage of an NPA over an OPA is that it can be used in either conscious or unconscious individuals because the device does not stimulate the gag reflex.

Advanced airway equipment includes the laryngeal mask airway, laryngeal tube, esophageal-tracheal tube, and endotracheal tube. Different styles of these supraglottic airways are available. If it is within your scope of practice, you may use advanced airway equipment when appropriate and available.

>> Next: Basic Airway Adjuncts

BASIC AIRWAY ADJUNCTS

OROPHARYNGEAL AIRWAY (OPA)

The OPA is a J-shaped device that fits over the tongue to hold the soft hypopharyngeal structures and the tongue away from the posterior wall of the pharynx. OPA is used in individuals who are at risk for developing airway obstruction from the tongue or from relaxed upper airway muscle. A properly sized and inserted OPA results in proper alignment with the glottis opening.

If efforts to open the airway fail to provide and maintain a clear, unobstructed airway, then use the OPA in unconscious persons. An OPA should not be used in a conscious or semiconscious individual, because it can stimulate gagging, vomiting, and possible aspiration. The key assessment to determine if an OPA can be placed is to check if the individual has an intact cough and gag reflex. If so, do not use an OPA.

NASOPHARYNGEAL AIRWAY (NPA)

The NPA is a soft rubber or plastic uncuffed tube that provides a conduit for airflow between the nares and the pharynx. It is used as an alternative to an OPA in individuals who need a basic airway management adjunct.

Unlike the oral airway, NPAs may be used in conscious or semiconscious individuals (individuals with intact cough and gag reflex). The NPA is indicated when insertion of an OPA is technically difficult or dangerous. NPA placement can be facilitated by the use of a lubricant. Never force placement of the NPA as severe nosebleeds may occur. If it does not fit in one nare, try the other side. Use caution or avoid placing NPAs in individuals with obvious facial fractures.

SUCTIONING

Suctioning is an essential component of maintaining a patent airway. Providers should suction the airway immediately if there are copious secretions, blood, or vomit. Attempts at suctioning should not exceed 10 seconds. To avoid hypoxemia, follow suctioning attempts with a short period of 100% oxygen administration.

Monitor the individual's heart rate, oxygen saturation, and clinical appearance during suctioning. If a change in monitoring parameters is seen, interrupt suctioning and administer oxygen until the heart rate returns to normal and until clinical condition improves. Assist ventilation as warranted.

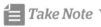 *Take Note*

- Only use an OPA in unresponsive individuals with NO cough or gag reflex. Otherwise, an OPA may stimulate vomiting, laryngeal spasm, or aspiration.

- An NPA can be used in conscious individuals with intact cough and gag reflex. However, use carefully in individuals with facial trauma due to the risk of displacement.

- Keep in mind that the individual is not receiving 100% oxygen while suctioning. Interrupt suctioning and administer oxygen if any deterioration in clinical picture is observed during suctioning.

>> Next: Basic Airway Technique

BASIC AIRWAY TECHNIQUE

INSERTING AN OPA

STEP 1: *Clear the mouth of blood and secretions with suction if possible.*

STEP 2: *Select an airway device that is the correct size for the person.*
- *Too large of an airway device can damage the throat.*
- *Too small of an airway device can press the tongue into the airway.*

STEP 3: *Place the device at the side of the person's face. Choose the device that extends from the corner of the mouth to the earlobe.*

STEP 4: *Insert the device into the mouth so the point is toward the roof of the mouth or parallel to the teeth.*
- *Do not press the tongue back into the throat.*

STEP 5: *Once the device is almost fully inserted, turn it until the tongue is cupped by the interior curve of the device.*

INSERTING AN NPA

STEP 1: *Select an airway device that is the correct size for the person.*

STEP 2: *Place the device at the side of the person's face. Choose the device that extends from the tip of the nose to the earlobe. Use the largest diameter device that will fit.*

STEP 3: *Lubricate the airway with a water-soluble lubricant or anesthetic jelly.*

STEP 4: *Insert the device slowly, moving straight into the face (not toward the brain).*

STEP 5: *It should feel snug; do not force the device into the nostril. If it feels stuck, remove it and try the other nostril.*

TIPS ON SUCTIONING

- When suctioning the oropharynx, do not insert the catheter too deeply. Extend the catheter to the maximum safe depth and suction as you withdraw.
- When suctioning an endotracheal (ET) tube, keep in mind the tube is within the trachea and that you may be suctioning near the bronchi or lung. Therefore, sterile technique should be used.
- Each suction attempt should be for no longer than 10 seconds. Remember the person will not get oxygen during suctioning.
- Monitor vital signs during suctioning and stop suctioning immediately if the person experiences hypoxemia (oxygen sats less than 94%), has a new arrhythmia or becomes cyanotic.

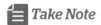 Take Note

- OPAs too large or too small may obstruct the airway.
- NPAs sized incorrectly may enter the esophagus.
- Always check for spontaneous respirations after insertion of either device.

>> Next: Advanced Airway Adjuncts

ADVANCED AIRWAY ADJUNCTS

ENDOTRACHEAL TUBE

The endotracheal (ET) tube is an advanced airway alternative. It is a specific type of tracheal tube that is inserted through the mouth or nose. It is the most technically difficult airway to place; however, it is the most secure airway available. Only experienced providers should perform ET intubation. This technique requires the use of a laryngoscope. Fiber optic portable laryngoscopes have a video screen, improve success, and are gaining popularity for field use.

LARYNGEAL MASK AIRWAY

The laryngeal mask airway (LMA) is an advanced airway alternative to ET intubation and provides comparable ventilation. It is acceptable to use the LMA as an alternative to an esophageal-tracheal tube for airway management in cardiac arrest. Experience will allow rapid placement of the LMA device by an ACLS provider.

LARYNGEAL TUBE

The advantages of the laryngeal tube are similar to those of the esophageal-tracheal tube; however, the laryngeal tube is more compact and less complicated to insert. This tube has only one larger balloon to inflate and can be inserted blindly.

ESOPHAGEAL-TRACHEAL TUBE

The esophageal-tracheal tube (sometimes referred to as a combitube) is an advanced airway alternative to ET intubation. This device provides adequate ventilation comparable to an ET tube. The combitube has two separate balloons that must be inflated and two separate ports. The provider must correctly determine which port to ventilate through to provide adequate oxygenation.

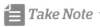 *Take Note*

- During CPR, the chest compression to ventilation rate is 30:2.
- If advanced airway is placed, do not interrupt chest compressions for breaths. Give one breath every 6 to 8 seconds.

>> Next: Routes of Access

ROUTES OF ACCESS

Historically in ACLS, providers have administered drugs via the intravenous (IV) or the ET route. ET absorption of drugs is poor, and optimal drug dosing is unknown. Therefore, the intraosseous (IO) route is now preferred when IV access is not available. Below are the priorities for vascular access.

INTRAVENOUS ROUTE

A peripheral IV is preferred for drug and fluid administration unless central line access is already available. Central line access is not necessary during most resuscitation attempts, as it may cause interruptions in CPR and complications during insertion. Placing a peripheral line does not require CPR interruption.

If a drug is given via peripheral route of administration, do the following:

1. Intravenously push bolus injection (unless otherwise indicated).

2. Flush with 20 mL of fluid or saline.

3. Raise extremity for 10 to 20 seconds to enhance delivery of drug to circulation.

INTRAOSSEOUS ROUTE

Drugs and fluids can be delivered safely and effectively during resuscitation via the IO route if IV access is not available.

IO access can be used for all age groups, can be placed in less than one minute, and has more predictable absorption than the ET route.

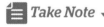 *Take Note*

- When using peripheral IV route of administration, drugs can take up to two minutes or more to reach central circulation. The effect of medications given may not be seen until even longer. High-quality CPR helps circulate these drugs and is an important part of resuscitation.

- Any ACLS drug or fluid that can be administered intravenously can also be given intraosseously.

>> Next: Pharmacological Tools

PHARMACOLOGICAL TOOLS

Use of any of the ALCS medication in Table 1 should be done within your scope of practice and after thorough study of the actions and side effects. This table only provides a brief reminder for those who are already knowledgeable in the use of these medications. Moreover, Table 1 contains only adult doses, indications, and routes of administration for the most common ACLS drugs.

Doses, Routes, and Uses of Common Drug

DRUG	MAIN ACLS USE	DOSE/ROUTE	NOTES
Adenosine	• *Narrow PSVT/SVT* • *Wide QRS tachycardia, avoid adenosine in irregular wide QRS*	• *6 mg IV bolus, may repeat with 12 mg in 1 to 2 min.*	• *Rapid IV push close to the hub, followed by a saline bolus* • *Continuous cardiac monitoring during administration* • *Causes flushing and chest heaviness*
Amiodarone	• *VF/pulseless VT* • *VT with pulse* • *Tachycardia rate control*	• *VF/VT: 300 mg dilute in 20 to 30 mL, may repeat 150 mg in 3 to 5 min*	• *Anticipate hypotension, bradycardia, and gastrointestinal toxicity* • *Continuous cardiac monitoring* • *Very long half-life (up to 40 days)* • *Do not use in 2nd or 3rd-degree heart block* • *Do not administer via the ET tube route*
Atropine	• *Symptomatic brady-cardia*	• *0.5 mg IV/IO every 3 to 5 minutes* • *Max dose: 3 mg*	• *Cardiac and BP monitoring* • *Do not use in glaucoma or tachyarrhythmias* • *Minimum dose 0.5 mg*
	• *Specific toxins/overdose (e.g. organophosphates)*	• *2 to 4 mg IV/IO may be needed*	
Dopamine	• *Shock/CHF*	• *2 to 20 mcg/kg/min* • *Titrate to desired blood pressure*	• *Fluid resuscitation first* • *Cardiac and BP monitoring*
Epinephrine	• *Cardiac Arrest*	• *Initial: 1.0 mg (1:10000) IV or 2 to 2.5 mg (1:1000) ET every 3 to 5 min* • *Maintain: 0.1 to 0.5 mcg/kg/min Titrate to desire blood pressure*	• *Continuous cardiac monitoring* • *Note: Distinguish between 1:1000 and 1:10000 concentrations* • *Give via central line when possible*
	• *Anaphylaxis*	• *0.3-0.5 mg IM* • *Repeat every five minutes as needed*	
	• *Symptomatic bradycardia/Shock*	• *2 to 10 mcg/min infusion* • *Titrate to response*	
Lidocaine (Lidocaine is recommended when Amiodarone is not available)	• *Cardiac Arrest (VF/VT)*	• *Initial: 1 to 1.5 mg/kg IV loading* • *Second: Half of first dose in 5 to 10 min* • *Maintain: 1 to 4 mg/min*	• *Cardiac and BP monitoring* • *Rapid bolus can cause hypotension and bradycardia* • *Use with caution in renal failure* • *Calcium chloride can reverse hypermagnesemia*
	• *Wide complex tachycardia with pulse*	• *Initial: 0.5 to 1.5 mg/kg IV* • *Second: Half of first dose in 5 to 10 min* • *Maintain: 1 to 4 mg/min*	
Magnesium Sulfate	• *Cardiac arrest/ Pulseless torsades*	• *Cardiac Arrest: 1 to 2 gm diluted in 10 mL D5W IVP*	• *Cardiac and BP monitoring* • *Rapid bolus can cause hypotension and bradycardia* • *Use with caution in renal failure* • *Calcium chloride can reverse hypermagne-semia*
	• *Torsades de Pointes with pulse*	• *If not cardiac arrest: 1 to 2 gm IV over 5 to 60 min Maintain: 0.5 to 1 gm/hr IV*	
Procainamide	• *Wide QRS tachycardia* • *Preferred for VT with pulse (stable)*	• *20 to 50 mg/min IV until rhythm improves, hypotension occurs, QRS widens by 50% or MAX dose is given* • *MAX dose: 17 mg/kg* • *Drip: 1 to 2 gm in 250 to 500 mL at 1 to 4 mg/min*	• *Cardiac and BP monitoring* • *Caution with acute MI* • *May reduce dose with renal failure* • *Do not give with amiodarone* • *Do not use in prolonged QT or CHF*
Sotalol	• *Tachyarrhythmia* • *Monomorphic VT* • *3rd line anti-arrhythmic*	• *100 mg (1.5 mg/kg) IV over 5 min*	• *Do not use in prolonged QT*

Table 1

>> Next: Self-Assessment for ACLS

1. An individual presents with symptomatic bradycardia. Her heart rate is 32. Which of the following are acceptable therapeutic options?

   a. Atropine
   b. Epinephrine
   c. Dopamine
   d. All of the above

2. A known alcoholic collapses and is found to be in Torsades de Pointes. What intervention is most likely to correct the underlying problem?

   a. Rewarm the individual to correct hypothermia.
   b. Administer magnesium sulfate 1 to 2 gm IV diluted in 10 mL D5W to correct low magnesium.
   c. Administer glucose to correct hypoglycemia.
   d. Administer naloxone to correct narcotic overdose.

3. You have just administered a drug for an individual in supraventricular tachycardia (SVT). She complains of flushing and chest heaviness. Which drug is the most likely cause?

   a. Aspirin
   b. Adenosine
   c. Amiodarone
   d. Amitriptyline

ANSWERS

1. D
   Atropine is the initial treatment for symptomatic bradycardia. If unresponsive, IV dopamine or epinephrine is the next step. Pacing may be effective if other measures fail to improve the rate.

2. B
   Hypomagnesemia or low Mg++ is commonly caused by alcoholism and malnutrition. Administration of IV magnesium may prevent or terminate torsades de pointes.

3. B
   Adenosine is the correct choice for SVT treatment and commonly results in reactions such as flushing, dyspnea, chest pressure, and lightheadedness.

>> Next: Principles of Early Defibrillation

PRINCIPLES OF EARLY DEFIBRILLATION

The earlier the defibrillation occurs, the higher the survival rate. When a fatal arrhythmia is present, CPR can provide a small amount of blood flow to the heart and the brain, but it cannot directly restore an organized rhythm. The likelihood of restoring a perfusing rhythm is optimized with immediate CPR and defibrillation. The purpose of defibrillation is to disrupt a chaotic rhythm and allow the heart's normal pacemakers to resume effective electrical activity.

The appropriate energy dose is determined by the design of the defibrillator—monophasic or biphasic. If you are using a monophasic defibrillator, give a single 360 J shock. Use the same energy dose on subsequent shocks. Biphasic defibrillators use a variety of waveforms and have been shown to be more effective for terminating a fatal arrhythmia. When using biphasic defibrillators, providers should use the manufacturer's recommended energy dose. Many biphasic defibrillator manufacturers display the effective energy dose range on the face of the device. If the first shock does not terminate the arrhythmia, it may be reasonable to escalate the energy delivered if the defibrillator allows it.

To minimize interruptions in chest compressions during CPR, continue CPR while the defibrillator is charging. Be sure to clear the individual by ensuring that oxygen is removed, and no one is touching the individual prior to delivering the shock. Immediately after the shock, resume CPR, beginning with chest compressions. Give CPR for two minutes (approximately five cycles). A cycle consists of 30 compressions followed by two breaths for an individual without an advanced airway. Those individuals with an advanced airway device in place can be ventilated at a rate of one breath every 5 to 6 seconds (or 10 to 12 breaths per minute).

>> *Next: Keys to Using an AED*

KEYS TO USING AN AUTOMATED EXTERNAL DEFIBRILLATOR

If you look around the public places you visit, you are likely to find an Automated External Defibrillator (AED). An AED is both sophisticated and easy to use, providing life-saving power in a user-friendly device which makes it useful for people who have never operated one and for anyone in stressful scenarios. However, proper use of an AED is very important.

Attach the pads to the upper right side and lower left side of the individual's chest *(Figure 11)*. Once the pads are attached correctly, the device will read the heart rhythm. If the pads are not attached appropriately, the device will indicate so with prompts. Once the rhythm is analyzed, the device will direct you to shock the individual if a shock is indicated. A shock depolarizes all heart muscle cells at once, attempting to organize its electrical activity. In other words, the shock is intended to reset the heart's abnormal electrical activity into a normal rhythm.

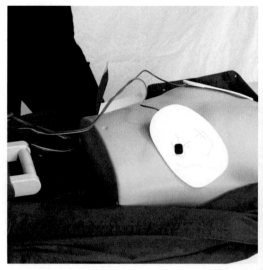

Figure 11

AED Key Points

Assure oxygen is NOT flowing across the patient's chest when delivering shock
Do NOT stop chest compressions for more than 10 seconds when assessing the rhythm
Stay clear of patient when delivering shock
Assess pulse after the first two minutes of CPR
If the end-tidal CO2 is less than 10 mmHg during CPR, consider adding a vasopressor and improve chest compressions

Figure 12

>> Next: Criteria to Apply AED

CRITERIA TO APPLY AED

You should use an AED if:

- The individual does not respond to shouting or shaking their shoulders.
- The individual is not breathing or breathing ineffectively.
- The carotid artery pulse cannot be detected.

BASIC AED OPERATION

To use an AED, do the following:

1. Power on the AED.
2. Choose adult or pediatric pads.
3. Attach the pads to bare chest (not over medication patches) and make sure cables are connected. (Dry the chest if necessary.)
4. Place one pad on upper right side and the other on the chest a few inches below the left arm.
5. Clear the area to allow AED to read rhythm, which may take up to 15 seconds.
6. If there is no rhythm in 15 seconds, restart CPR.
7. If the AED indicates a shock is needed, clear the individual, making sure no one is touching them and that the oxygen has been removed. Ensure visually that the individual is clear and shout "CLEAR!"
8. Press the "Shock" button.
9. Immediately resume CPR starting with chest compressions.
10. After two minutes of CPR, analyze the rhythm with the AED.
11. Continue to follow the AED prompts.

 Take Note

- If the AED is not working properly, continue CPR. Do not waste excessive time troubleshooting the AED. CPR always comes first, and AEDs are supplemental.

- Do not use the AED in water.

- AED is not contraindicated in individuals with implanted defibrillator/ pacemaker; however, do not place pad directly over the device.

>> Next: Systems of Care

6 SYSTEMS OF CARE

The AHA guidelines describe Systems of Care as a separate and important part of ACLS provider training. These Systems of Care describe the organization of professionals necessary to achieve the best possible result for a given individual's circumstances. They include an overview of the ways life-saving interventions should be organized to ensure they are delivered efficiently and effectively. Hospitals, EMS staff, and communities that follow comprehensive Systems of Care demonstrate better outcomes for their patients than those who do not.

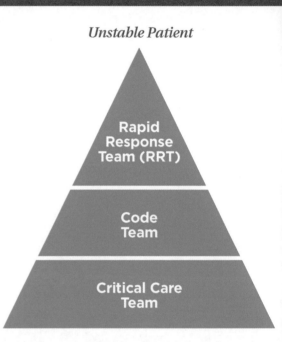

Unstable Patient

Rapid Response Team (RRT)

Code Team

Critical Care Team

Figure 13

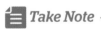 *Take Note*

- Management of life-threatening emergencies requires the integration of a multidisciplinary team that can involve rapid response teams (RRTs), cardiac arrest teams, and intensive care specialists to increase survival rates.

- 2015 guidelines update reflects research that shows that RRTs improve outcomes.

>> Next: Cardiopulmonary Resuscitation

CARDIOPULMONARY RESUSCITATION

Successful cardiopulmonary resuscitation (CPR) requires the use of it as part of a system of care called the Chain of Survival *(Figure 14)*. As with any chain, it is only as strong as its weakest link. Thus, everyone must strive to make sure each link is strong. For instance, community leaders can work to increase awareness of the signs and symptoms of cardiac arrest and make AEDs available in public places. EMS crews must stay abreast of updates and innovations in resuscitation and hone the skills required to deliver CPR quickly and effectively. Hospitals should be ready to receive patients in cardiac arrest and provide excellent care. Critical care and reperfusion centers should be staffed by experts and equipped with the latest technology.

INITIATING THE CHAIN OF SURVIVAL

Early initiation of BLS has been shown to increase the probability of survival for a person dealing with cardiac arrest. To increase the odds of surviving a cardiac event, the rescuer should follow the steps in the Adult Chain of Survival *(Figure 14)*.

Adult Chain of Survival

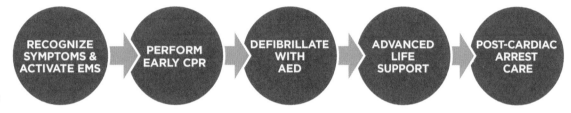

Figure 14

>> Next: Post-Cardiac Arrest Care

POST-CARDIAC ARREST CARE

Integrated post-cardiac arrest care is the last link in the Adult Chain of Survival. The quality of this care is critical to providing resuscitated individuals with the best possible results. When the interventions below are provided, there is an increased likelihood of survival.

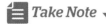

Take Note

> The 2015 guidelines update recommends a focused debriefing of rescuers/providers for the purpose of performance improvement.

THERAPEUTIC HYPOTHERMIA

- Recommended for comatose individuals with return of spontaneous circulation after a cardiac arrest event.
- Individuals should be cooled to 89.6 to 93.2 degrees F (32 to 36 degrees C) for at least 24 hours.

OPTIMIZATION OF HEMODYNAMICS AND VENTILATION

- 100% oxygen is acceptable for early intervention but not for extended periods of time.
- Oxygen should be titrated, so that individual's pulse oximetry is greater than 94% to avoid oxygen toxicity.
- Do not over ventilate to avoid potential adverse hemodynamic effects.
- Ventilation rates of 10 to 12 breaths per minute to achieve ETCO2 at 35 to 40 mmHg.
- IV fluids and vasoactive medications should be titrated for hemodynamic stability.

PERCUTANEOUS CORONARY INTERVENTION

- Percutaneous coronary intervention (PCI) is preferred over thrombolytics.
- Individual should be taken by EMS directly to a hospital that performs PCI.
- If the individual is delivered to a center that only delivers thrombolytics, they should be transferred to a center that offers PCI if time permits.

NEUROLOGICAL CARE

- Neurologic assessment is key, especially when withdrawing care (i.e., brain death) to decrease false-positive rates. Specialty consultation should be obtained to monitor neurologic signs and symptoms throughout the post-resuscitation period.

>> Next: Acute Coronary Syndrome

ACUTE CORONARY SYNDROME

For individuals with acute coronary syndrome (ACS), proper care starts during the call to EMS. First responders must be aware of and look for signs of ACS. Quick diagnosis and treatment yield the best chance to preserve healthy heart tissue. It is very important that health care providers recognize individuals with potential ACS in order to initiate evaluation, appropriate triage, and time management.

STEMI Chain of Survival

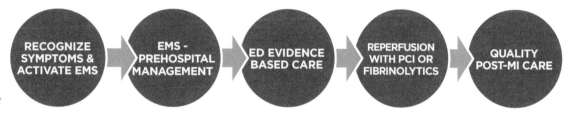

Figure 15

GOALS OF ACS TREATMENT

Early EMS communication allows for preparation of emergency department personnel and cardiac catheterization lab and staff. Once the ACS patient arrives at the receiving facility, established protocols should direct care. The shorter the time is until reperfusion, the greater the amount of heart tissue that can be saved, and the more optimal the overall outcome.

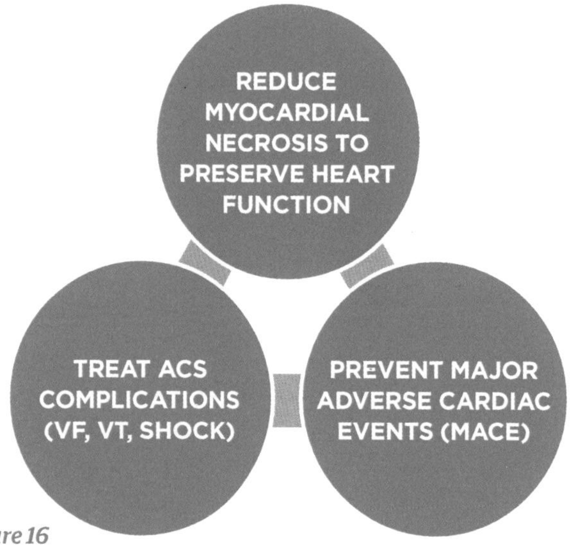

Major adverse cardiac events (MACE) includes death and non-fatal myocardial infarction. Life-threatening complications of ACS include ventricular fibrillation, pulseless ventricular tachycardia, bradyarrhythmias, cardiogenic shock, and pulmonary edema. EMS should have the capacity to perform ECGs on scene and on the way to the hospital. The receiving hospital should be made aware of possible ACS, especially ST-elevation myocardial infarction elevation (STEMI) and non-ST-elevation myocardial infarction (NSTEMI).

Figure 16

>> Next: Acute Stroke

ACUTE STROKE

Outcomes for individuals with stroke have improved significantly due to the implementation of Acute Stroke System of Care. The community is better equipped to recognize stroke as a "brain attack," and there is greater awareness of the importance of medical care within one hour of symptom onset. Likewise, EMS systems have been enhanced to transport individuals to regional stroke care centers that are equipped to administer fibrinolytics.

Stroke Chain of Survival

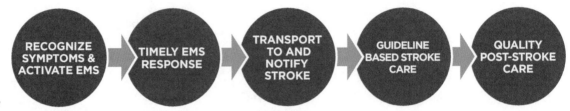

Figure 17

GOALS OF ACUTE ISCHEMIC STROKE CARE

The overall goal of stroke care is to minimize brain injury and optimize the individual's recovery. Preferential transport to stroke-capable centers has been shown to improve outcomes. Stroke centers are equipped with resources often not available at smaller community hospitals. The presence of specialists, including neurologists and stroke care specialists, multidisciplinary teams experienced in stroke care, advanced imaging modalities, and other therapeutic options make transport to stroke centers the most suitable option. The goal of the stroke team, emergency physician, or other experts should be to assess the individual with suspected stroke within ten minutes.

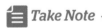 *Take Note*

> The 8 D's of Stroke Care (Table 2) highlight the major steps of diagnosis and treatment of stroke and key points at which delays can occur.

The 8 D's of Stroke Care

DETECTION	*Rapid recognition of stroke systems*
DISPATCH	*Early activation and dispatch of EMS by 911*
DELIVERY	*Rapid EMS identification, management, and transport*
DOOR	*Transport to stroke center*
DATA	*Rapid triage, evaluation, and management in ED*
DECISION	*Stroke expertise and therapy selection*
DRUG	*Fibrinolytic therapy, intra-arterial strategies*
DISPOSITION	*Rapid admission to the stroke unit or critical care unit*

Table 2

>> Next: The Resuscitation Team

THE RESUSCITATION TEAM

The AHA guidelines for ACLS highlight the importance of effective team dynamics during resuscitation. In the community (outside a health care facility), the first rescuer on the scene may be performing CPR alone. However, a Code Blue in a hospital may bring dozens of responders/providers to a patient's room. It is important to quickly and efficiently organize team members to effectively participate in ACLS. The AHA suggests a team structure with each provider assuming a specific role during the resuscitation; this consists of a team leader and several team members see *(Table 3)*.

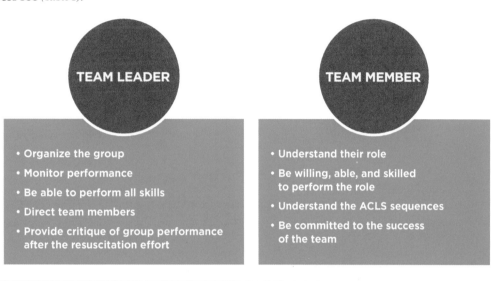

TEAM LEADER

- Organize the group
- Monitor performance
- Be able to perform all skills
- Direct team members
- Provide critique of group performance after the resuscitation effort

TEAM MEMBER

- Understand their role
- Be willing, able, and skilled to perform the role
- Understand the ACLS sequences
- Be committed to the success of the team

Table 3

 Take Note

Clear communication between team leaders and team members is essential.

It is important to know your own clinical limitations. Resuscitation is the time for implementing acquired skills, not trying new ones. Only take on tasks you can perform successfully. Clearly state when you need help and call for help early in the care of the individual. Resuscitation demands mutual respect, knowledge sharing, constructive criticism, and follow-up discussion (debriefing) after the event.

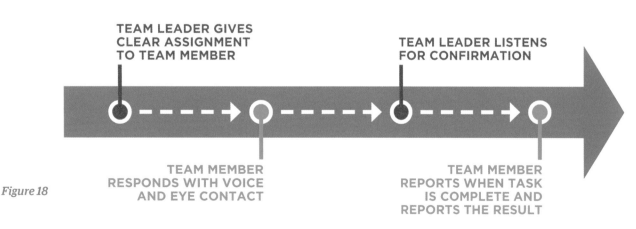

TEAM LEADER GIVES CLEAR ASSIGNMENT TO TEAM MEMBER

TEAM LEADER LISTENS FOR CONFIRMATION

TEAM MEMBER RESPONDS WITH VOICE AND EYE CONTACT

TEAM MEMBER REPORTS WHEN TASK IS COMPLETE AND REPORTS THE RESULT

Figure 18

>> Next: Education, Implementation, Teams

EDUCATION, IMPLEMENTATION, TEAMS

Only about 20% of the individuals who have a cardiac arrest inside a hospital will survive. This statistic prompted the development of a Cardiac Arrest System of Care. Four out of five individuals with cardiopulmonary arrest have changes in vital signs prior to the arrest. Therefore, most individuals who eventually have a cardiac arrest showed signs of impending cardiac arrest. Survival rate could be improved if individuals are identified and treated with ACLS protocols sooner.

Originally, specialized groups of responders within a hospital, called Cardiac Arrest Teams, attended to a patient with recognized cardiac arrest. These teams responded to a Code Blue after someone presumably recognized an active cardiac arrest and sought help. Many believed Cardiac Arrest Teams would improve survival rates, but the results were disappointing. Studies show that survival rates were the same in hospitals with Cardiac Arrest Teams as in those without a team. As a result, hospitals are replacing Cardiac Arrest Teams with Rapid Response Teams (RRTs) or Medical Emergency Teams (METs).

Rather than waiting for loss of consciousness and full cardiopulmonary arrest, RRTs/METs closely monitor patients in order to treat them before the cardiac arrest occurs. These teams combine the efforts of nurses, physicians, and family members to detect an impending cardiac arrest.

RRT/MET ALERT CRITERIA

THREATENED AIRWAY OR LABORED BREATHING	ALTERED MENTAL STATUS
BRADYCARDIA (< 40 BPM) OR TACHYCARDIA (> 100 BPM)	SEIZURE
HYPOTENSION OR SYMPTOMATIC HYPERTENSION	SUDDEN AND LARGE DECREASE IN URINE OUTPUT

Figure 19

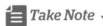 *Take Note*

When hospitals implement RRTs/METs, there are fewer cardiac arrests, fewer ICU transfers, improved survival rates, and shorter length of inpatient stay.

>> *Next: Self-Assessment for Systems of Care*

SELF-ASSESSMENT FOR SYSTEMS OF CARE

1. What is the longest a rescuer should pause to check for a pulse?

    a. 20 seconds
    b. 10 seconds
    c. 5 seconds
    d. Less than two seconds

2. Select the proper pairing regarding CPR:

    a. Chest compressions 60 to 80/minute; 2 inches deep
    b. Chest compressions 80/minute; 1.5 inches deep
    c. Chest compressions 100/minute; 3 inches deep
    d. Chest compression 100 to 120 per minute; 2 to 2.4 inches deep

3. What is the role of the second rescuer during a cardiac arrest scenario?

    a. Summon help.
    b. Retrieve AED.
    c. Perform ventilations.
    d. All of the above

ANSWERS

1. B
   Pulse checks are limited to no more than 10 seconds. If you are unsure whether a pulse is present, begin CPR.

2. D
   Compress the adult chest two inches at a rate of at least 100 per minute.

3. D
   Take advantage of any bystander and enlist their help based on their skill level.

>> Next: ACLS Cases

7

ACLS CASES

RESPIRATORY ARREST

Individuals with ineffective breathing patterns are considered to be in respiratory arrest and require immediate attention. There are many causes of respiratory arrest, including but not limited to cardiac arrest and cardiogenic shock. Resuscitate individuals in apparent respiratory arrest using either the BLS or the ACLS Survey.

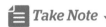 *Take Note*

Respiratory arrest is an emergent condition in which the individual is either not breathing or is breathing ineffectively.

>> Next: BLS Survey

BLS Survey

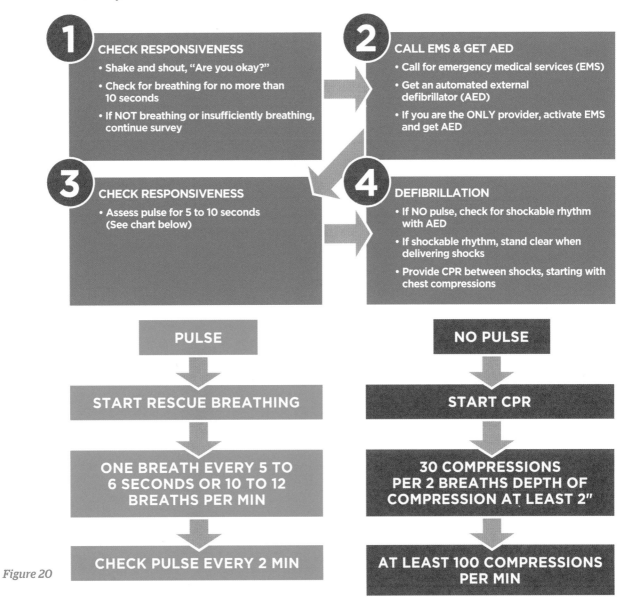

Figure 20

>> *Next: ACLS Survey*

ACLS Survey

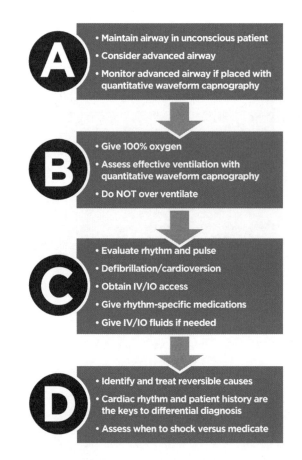

Figure 21

TYPES OF VENTILATION

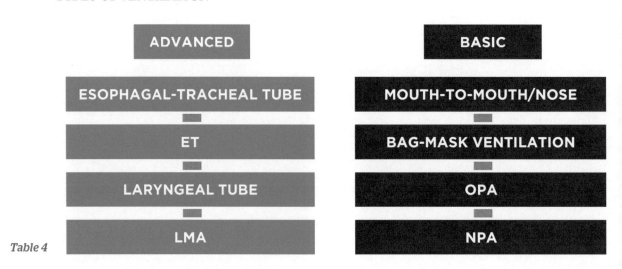

Table 4

>> *Next: Types of Ventilation*

In Table 4, the airways listed in the left column are considered advanced airways, while those in the right column are basic airways. Although OPAs and NPAs are considered to be basic airways, they require proper placement by an experienced provider. Advanced airway insertion requires specialized training beyond the scope of ACLS certification. While the placement of advanced airways require specialized training, all ACLS providers should know the proper use of advanced airways once they are placed. Regardless of airway type, proper airway management is an important part of ACLS.

CPR is performed with the individual lying on their back; gravity will cause the jaw, the tongue, and the tissues of the throat to fall back and obstruct the airway. The airway rarely remains open in an unconscious individual without external support.

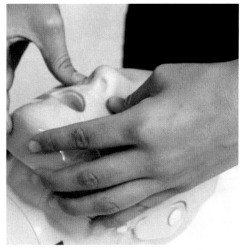

Figure 22

The first step in any airway intervention is to open the airway. This is accomplished by lifting the chin upward while tilting the forehead back *(Figure 22)*. The goal is to create a straighter path from the nose to the trachea.

In individuals with suspected neck injury, the cervical spine should be protected and a jaw thrust alone is used to open the airway *(Figure 23)*. While the standard practice in a suspected neck injury is to place a cervical collar, this should not be done in BLS or ACLS. Cervical collars can compress the airway and interfere with resuscitation efforts. The provider must ensure an open airway regardless of the basic airway used. The provider is obligated to stabilize the head or ask for assistance while maintaining control of the airway.

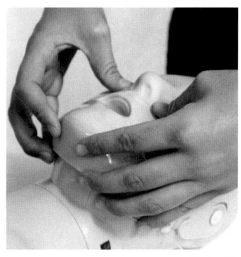

Figure 23

 Take Note

> Do not over ventilate (i.e., give too many breaths per minute or too large volume per breath). Both can increase intrathoracic pressure, decrease venous return to heart, diminish cardiac output, as well as predispose individuals to vomit and aspiration of gastrointestinal contents.

>> *Next: Ventricular Fibrillation and Pulseless Ventricular Tachycardia*

VENTRICULAR FIBRILLATION AND PULSELESS VENTRICULAR TACHYCARDIA

Ventricular fibrillation (VF) and pulseless ventricular tachycardia (VT) are life-threatening cardiac rhythms that result in ineffective ventricular contractions. VF *(Figure 24)* is a rapid quivering of the ventricular walls that prevents them from pumping. The ventricular motion of VF is not synchronized with atrial contractions. VT *(Figure 25)* is a condition in which the ventricles contract more than 100 times per minute. The emergency condition, pulseless VT, occurs when ventricular contraction is so rapid that there is no time for the heart to refill, resulting in undetectable pulse. In both cases, individuals are not receiving adequate blood flow to the tissues. Despite being different pathological phenomena and having different ECG rhythms, the ACLS management of VF and VT are essentially the same. Resuscitation for VF and pulseless VT starts with the BLS Survey.

An AED reads and analyzes the rhythm and determines if a shock is needed. The AED is programmed to only prompt the user to shock VF and VT rhythms. The machine does not know if the individual has a pulse or not. This is the primary reason you should not use an AED in someone with a palpable pulse. ACLS responses to VF and pulseless VT within a hospital will likely be conducted using a cardiac monitor and a manual defibrillator. Thus, the ACLS provider must read and analyze the rhythm. Shocks should only be delivered for VF and pulseless VT. Likewise, antiarrhythmic drugs and drugs to support blood pressure may be used.

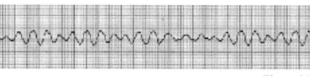

Figure 24

RULES FOR VENTRICULAR FIBRILLATION (VF)

REGULARITY	*There is no regularity shape of the QRS complex because all electrical activity is disorganized.*
RATE	*The rate appears rapid, but the disorganized electrical activity prevents the heart from pumping.*
P WAVE	*There are no P waves present.*
PR INTERVAL	*There are no PR intervals present.*
QRS COMPLEX	*The ventricle complex varies*

Table 5

>> *Next: Rules for Ventricular Tachycardia*

RULES FOR
VENTRICULAR TACHYCARDIA
(REGULAR/RAPID WIDE
COMPLEX TACHYCARDIA)

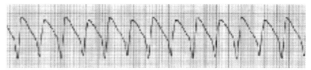

Figure 25

REGULARITY	*R-R intervals are usually, but not always, regular.*
RATE	*The atrial rate cannot be determined. Ventricular rate is usually between 150 and 250 beats per minute.*
P WAVE	*QRS complexes are not preceded by P waves. There are occasionally P waves in the strip, but they are not associated with the ventricular rhythm.*
PR INTERVAL	*PR interval is not measured since this is a ventricular rhythm.*
QRS COMPLEX	*QRS complex measures more than 0.12 seconds. The QRS will usually be wide and bizarre. It is usually difficult to see a separation between the QRS complex and the T wave.*

Table 6

RULES FOR
TORSADES DE POINTES
(IRREGULAR WIDE
COMPLEX TACHYCARDIA)

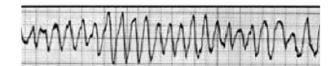

Figure 26

REGULARITY	*There is no regularity.*
RATE	*The atrial rate cannot be determined. Ventricular rate is usually between 150 and 250 beats per minute.*
P WAVE	*There are no P waves present.*
PR INTERVAL	*There are no PR intervals present.*
QRS COMPLEX	*The ventricle complex varies.*

Table 7

 Take Note

VF and pulseless VT are both shockable rhythms. The AED cannot tell if the individual has a pulse or not.

>> Next: Pulseless Electrical Activity and Asystole

PULSELESS ELECTRICAL ACTIVITY AND ASYSTOLE

Pulseless electrical activity (PEA) and asystole are related cardiac rhythms in that they are both life-threatening and unshockable. Asystole is a flat-line ECG *(Figure 27)*. There may be subtle movement away from baseline (drifting flat-line), but there is no perceptible cardiac electrical activity. Always ensure that a reading of asystole is not a user or technical error. Make sure patches have good contact with the individual, leads are connected, gain is set appropriately, and the power is on. PEA is one of many waveforms by ECG (including sinus rhythm) without a detectable pulse. PEA may include any pulseless waveform with the exception of VF, VT, or asystole.

Hypovolemia and hypoxia are the two most common causes of PEA. They are also the most easily reversible and should be at the top of any differential diagnosis.

If the individual has return of spontaneous circulation (ROSC), proceed to post-cardiac arrest care. Atropine is no longer recommended in cases of PEA or asystole.

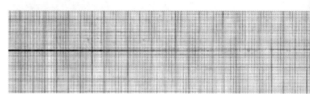

Figure 27

RULES FOR PEA AND ASYSTOLE

REGULARITY	*The rhythm will be a nearly flat line.*
RATE	*There is no rate.*
P WAVE	*There are no P waves present.*
PR INTERVAL	*PR interval is unable to be measured due to no P waves being present.*
QRS COMPLEX	*There are no QRS complexes present.*

Table 8

>> Next: Reversible Causes

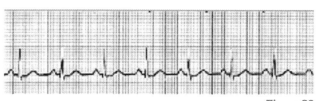

REVERSIBLE CAUSES

Figure 28

REVERSIBLE CAUSES OF CARDIAC ARREST	
THE H'S	**THE T'S**
Hypovolemia	Tension pneumothorax
Hypoxia	Tamponade
H+ (acidosis)	Toxins
Hypo/Hyperkalemia	Thrombosis (coronary)
Hypoglycemia	Thrombosis (pulmonary)
Hypothermia	Trauma (unrecognized)

Table 9

 Take Note

• Always verify that a reading of asystole is not equipment failure. Make sure patches make good contact with the individual, all cables are connected, gain is set appropriately, and the power is on.

• Hypovolemia and hypoxia are easily reversed and are the two most common causes of PEA.

NO ATROPINE DURING PEA OR ASYSTOLE

Although there is no evidence that atropine has a detrimental effect during bradycardia or asystolic cardiac arrest, routine use of atropine during PEA or asystole has not been shown to have a therapeutic benefit. Therefore, the AHA has removed atropine from the cardiac arrest guidelines.

STANDARD DOSE EPINEPHRINE IS VASOPRESSOR OF CHOICE

Preliminary research suggested that epinephrine in higher doses may produce improved results in resuscitation. However, research conducted after the 2010 guidelines publication failed to show any benefit over standard dose of 1 mg epinephrine. Likewise, the 2010 AHA guidelines offered an alternative vasopressor, called vasopressin, which could be used instead of or after the first dose of epinephrine. Subsequent research showed that vasopressin offered no benefit over standard dose epinephrine. Without a demonstration of superiority, both high-dose epinephrine and vasopressin have been removed, simplifying the ACLS algorithm.

>> Next: Adult Cardiac Arrest Algorithm

Adult Cardiac Arrest Algorithm

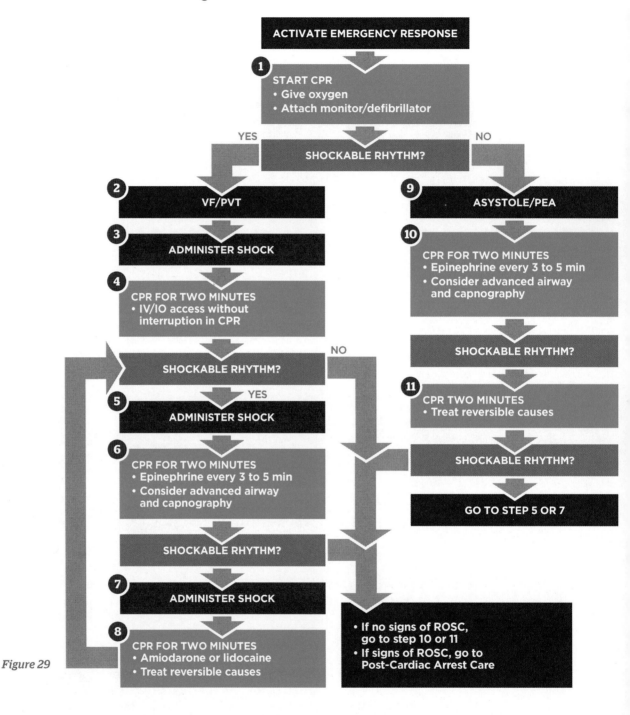

Figure 29

>> Next: Adult Cardiac Arrest Algorithm Continued

ADULT CARDIAC ARREST ALGORITHM CONTINUED

CPR Quality

- Push hard (≥ 2 inches) and fast (≥ 100 bpm) and allow chest recoil
- Minimize interruptions
- Do not over ventilate
- If no advanced airway, 30:2 compression to ventilation ratio
- Quantitative waveform capnography
    - If ETCO2 <10 mmHg, attempt to improve CPR quality
- Intra-arterial pressure
    - If diastolic pressure < 20 mmHg, attempt to improve CPR quality

Shock Energy

- Biphasic: Biphasic delivery of energy during defibrillation has been shown to be more effective than older monophasic waveforms. Follow manufacturer recommendation (e.g., initial dose of 120 to 200 J); if unknown, use maximumly available. Second and subsequent doses should be equivalent and higher doses should be considered.
- Monophasic: 360 J

Return of Spontaneous Circulation

- Return of pulse and blood pressure
- Sudden sustained increase in PETCO2 (typically ≥ 40 mmHg)
- Spontaneous arterial pressure waves with intra-arterial monitoring

Advanced Airway

- Supraglottic advanced airway or ET intubation
- Waveform capnography to confirm and monitor ET tube placement
- 8 to 10 breaths per minute with continuous chest compressions

Drug Therapy

- Epinephrine IV/IO Dose: 1 mg every 3 to 5 minutes
- Amiodarone IV/IO Dose: first dose is 300 mg bolus, second dose is 150 mg

Reversible Causes

- Hypovolemia
- Hypoxia
- H+(acidosis)
- Hypothermia
- Hypo-/hyperkalemia
- Tamponade, cardiac
- Toxins
- Tension pneumothorax
- Thrombosis, pulmonary or coronary

>> Next: Post-Cardiac Arrest Care

POST-CARDIAC ARREST CARE

If an individual has a return of spontaneous circulation (ROSC), start post-cardiac arrest care immediately. The initial BLS/ACLS processes are meant to save an individual's life, while post-cardiac arrest care is meant to optimize ventilation and circulation, preserve heart and brain tissue/function, and maintain recommended blood glucose levels.

BLOOD PRESSURE SUPPORT AND VASOPRESSORS

- Consider blood pressure support in any individual with systolic blood pressure less than 90 mmHg or mean arterial pressure (MAP) less than 65.
- Unless contraindicated, 1 to 2 liters of IV saline or Lactated Ringer's is the first intervention.
- When blood pressure is very low, consider vasopressors (commonly referred to as "pressors"):
- If no advanced airway, 30:2 compression to ventilation ratio
    - Epinephrine is the pressor of choice for individuals who are not in cardiac arrest.
    - Dopamine, phenylephrine, and methoxamine are alternatives to epinephrine.
    - Norepinephrine is generally reserved for severe hypotension or as a last-line agent.
- Titrate the infusion rate to maintain the desired blood pressure.

HYPOTHERMIA

Hypothermia is the only documented intervention that improves/enhances brain recovery after cardiac arrest. It can be performed in unresponsive individuals (i.e., comatose) and should be continued for at least 24 hours. The goal of induced hypothermia is to maintain a core body temperature between 89.6 to 93.2 degrees F (32 to 36 degrees C). Device manufacturers have developed several innovative technologies that improve the ability to affect and manage hypothermia in the post-arrest individual. Hypothermia should be induced and monitored by trained professionals. Induced hypothermia should not affect the decision to perform percutaneous coronary intervention (PCI), because concurrent PCI and hypothermia are reported to be feasible and safe.

>> Next: Adult Immediate Post-Cardiac Arrest Care Algorithm

Adult Immediate Post-Cardiac Arrest Care Algorithm

VENTILATION/OXYGENATION:
Avoid excessive ventilation. Start at 10 to 12 breaths per minute and titrate to target PETCO2 of 35 to 40 mmHg.

DOSES/DETAILS

IV Bolus:
1 to 2 liters normal saline or Lactated Ringer's. If inducing hypothermia, consider 4°C fluid.

Epinephrine IV Infusion:
0.1 to 0.5 mcg/kg per minute

Dopamine IV Infusion:
5 to 10 mcg/kg per minute

Norepinephrine IV Infusion:
0.1 to 0.5 mcg/kg per minute

REVERSIBLE CAUSES:

- Hypovolemia
- Hypoxia
- H+ (acidosis)
- Hypothermia
- Hypo-/hyperkalemia
- Tamponade, cardiac
- Toxins
- Tension pneumothorax
- Thrombosis, pulmonary

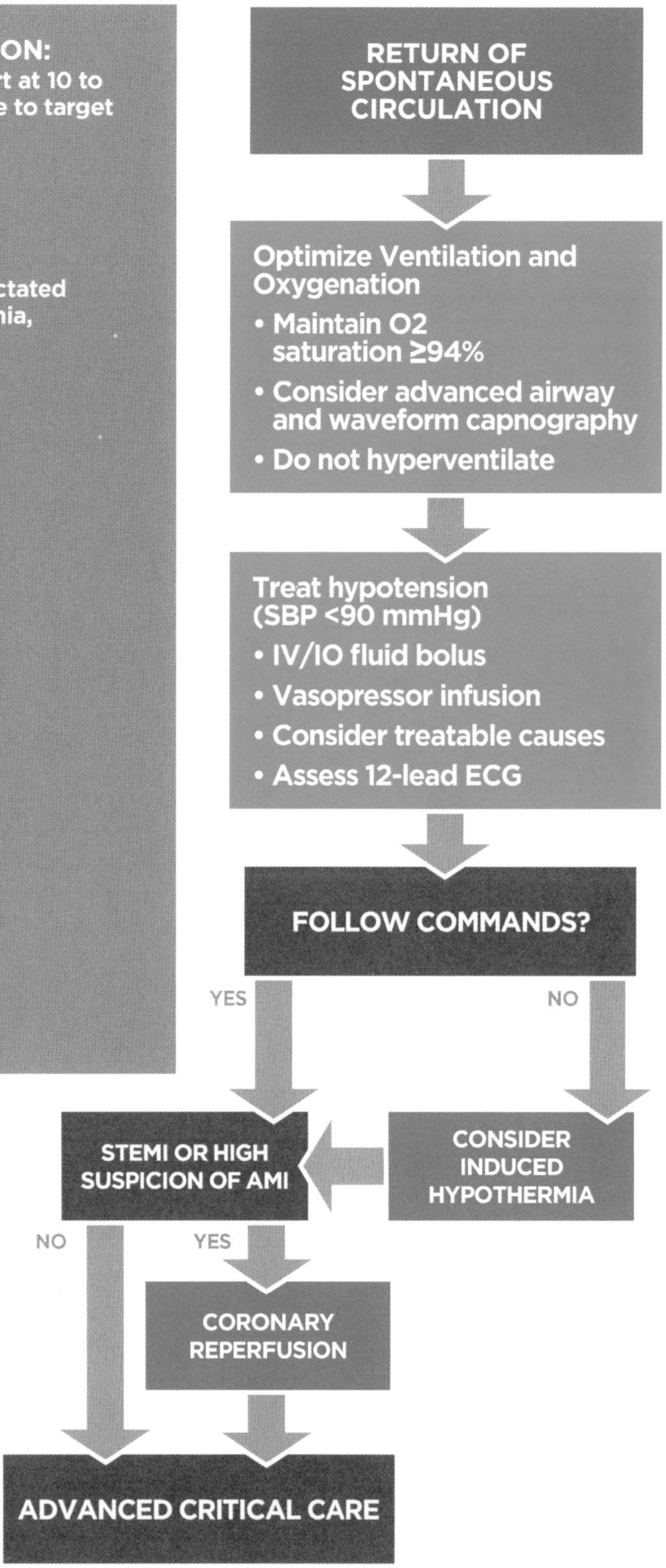

RETURN OF SPONTANEOUS CIRCULATION

↓

Optimize Ventilation and Oxygenation
- Maintain O2 saturation ≥94%
- Consider advanced airway and waveform capnography
- Do not hyperventilate

↓

Treat hypotension (SBP <90 mmHg)
- IV/IO fluid bolus
- Vasopressor infusion
- Consider treatable causes
- Assess 12-lead ECG

↓

FOLLOW COMMANDS?

YES | NO

STEMI OR HIGH SUSPICION OF AMI ← **CONSIDER INDUCED HYPOTHERMIA**

NO | YES

CORONARY REPERFUSION

ADVANCED CRITICAL CARE

Figure 30

>> *Next: Symptomatic Bradycardia*

RULES FOR SINUS BRADYCARDIA

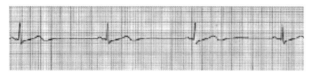

Figure 31

REGULARITY	R-R intervals are regular, overall rhythm is regular.
RATE	The rate is less than 60 bpm, but usually more than 40 bpm.
P WAVE	There is one P wave in front of every QRS. The P waves appear uniform.
PR INTERVAL	Measures between 0.12 and 0.20 seconds in duration. PRI is consistent.
QRS COMPLEX	Measures less than 0.12 seconds.

Table 10 & 11

RULES FOR FIRST DEGREE

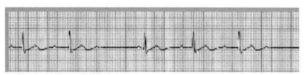

Figure 32

REGULARITY	R-R intervals are regular, overall rhythm is regular.
RATE	The rate depends on the underlying rhythm.
P WAVE	There is one P wave in front of every QRS. The P waves appear uniform.
PR INTERVAL	Measures more than 0.20 seconds in duration. PR interval is consistent.
QRS COMPLEX	Measures less than 0.12 seconds.

RULES FOR 2ND DEGREE TYPE I AV BLOCK (WENCKEBACH)

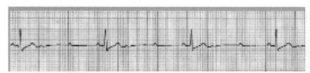

Figure 33

REGULARITY	R-R interval is irregular, but there is usually a pattern to it. The R-R interval gets longer as the PR interval gets longer.
RATE	The ventricular rate is usually slightly higher than the atrial rate due to some atrial beats not being conducted. The atrial rate is usually normal.
P WAVE	P waves are upright and uniform. Most complexes will have a P wave in front of them; however, there will be some that do not have a P wave.
PR INTERVAL	PR interval gets progressively longer until there is a dropped QRS complex.
QRS COMPLEX	Measures less than 0.12 seconds.

Table 12 & 13

RULES FOR 2ND DEGREE TYPE II AV BLOCK (MOBITZ II)

Figure 34

REGULARITY	If there is a consistent conduction ratio, then the R-R interval will be regular. If the conduction ratio is not constant, the R-R interval will be irregular.
RATE	The atrial rate is normal. The ventricular rate is slower, usually 1/2 to 1/3, slower than the atrial rate.
P WAVE	P waves are upright and uniform. There is not a QRS following every P wave.
PR INTERVAL	PR interval can only be measured on conducted beats, and it is usually constant across the strip. It may or may not be longer than a normal PR interval (0.12 seconds).
QRS COMPLEX	Measures less than 0.12 seconds.

>> Next: Rules for 3rd Degree AV Block

*RULES FOR 3RD
DEGREE AV BLOCK
(COMPLETE HEART BLOCK)*

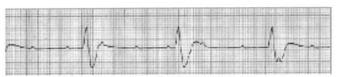

Figure 35

REGULARITY	*R-R interval is regular. P-P interval is also regular.*
RATE	*The atrial rate is regular and normally 60 to 100. Rate of QRS complexes is dependent on the focus.* *If the focus is ventricular, the rate will be 20 to 40.* *If the focus is junctional, the rate will be 40 to 60.*
P WAVE	*P waves are upright and uniform. There is not a QRS following every P wave.*
PR INTERVAL	*PR interval can only be measured on conducted beats, and it is usually constant across the strip. It may or may not be longer than a normal PR interval (0.12 seconds).*
QRS COMPLEX	*Interval may be normal but is more likely to be prolonged.*

Table 14

SYMPTOMATIC BRADYCARDIA

Bradycardia is defined as a heart rate of less than 60 beats per minute. While any heart rate less than 60 beats per minute is considered bradycardia, not every individual with bradycardia is symptomatic or having a pathological event. Individuals in excellent physical shape often have sinus bradycardia. Symptomatic bradycardia may cause a number of signs and symptoms including low blood pressure, pulmonary edema, and congestion, abnormal rhythm, chest discomfort, shortness of breath, lightheadedness, and/or confusion. Symptomatic bradycardia should be treated with the ACLS Survey. If bradycardia is asymptomatic but occurs with an arrhythmia listed below, obtain a consultation from a cardiologist experienced in treating rhythm disorders.

SYMPTOMS OF BRADYCARDIA

- Shortness of breath
- Altered mental status
- Hypotension
- Pulmonary edema/congestion
- Weakness/dizziness/lightheadedness

>> Next: Symptomatic Bradycardia Review

SYMPTOMATIC BRADYCARDIA REVIEW

Sinus Bradycardia

- Normal rhythm with slow rate

First Degree AV Block

- PR interval is longer than 0.20 seconds

Type I Second Degree AV Block

- PR interval increases in length until QRS complex is dropped

Type II Second Degree AV Block

- PR interval is the same length until intermittently dropped QRS complex is dropped

Third Degree AV Block

- PR and QRS are not coordinated with each other

>> Next: Adult Bradycardia with Pulse Algorithm

Adult Bradycardia with Pulse Algorithm

Assess signs/symptoms
Heart rate typically <50
beats per minute if
bradyarrhythmia

IDENTIFY AND TREAT
UNDERLYING CAUSE:

- **Maintain patent airway; assist breathing if necessary**
- **If hypoxemic, administer oxygen**
- **Cardiac monitor to identify rhythm**
- **Monitor blood pressure and pulse oximetry**
- **IV access**
- **Assess 12-lead ECG**

PERSISTENT
BRADYARRHYHMIA CAUSING:

- **Hypotension?**
- **Acutely altered mental status?**
- **Signs of shock?**
- **Chest pain?**
- **Acute heart failure?**

NO →

MONITOR AND OBSERVE

ATROPINE *(See Doses/Details)*
IF ATROPINE INEFFECTIVE:

- **Transcutaneous pacing**

OR

- **Dopamine infusion: 2 to 10 mcg/kg per minute**

OR

- **Epinephrine infusion: 2 to 10 mcg per minute**

CONSIDER:

- **Specialist consultation**
- **Transvenous pacing**

VENTILATION/OXYGENATION:

Avoid excessive ventilation. Start at 10 to 12 breaths/min and titrate to target PETCO2 of 35 to 40 mmHg

DOSES/DETAILS

Atropine IV Dose:

Initial dose of 0.5 mg bolus.

Repeat every 3 to 5 minutes up to 3 mg max dose

Dopamine IV infusion:

2 to 20 mcg/kg per minute. Titrate to patient response; taper slowly.

Epinephrine IV infusion:

5 to 10 mcg per minute

Figure 36

>> Next: Tachycardia

TACHYCARDIA

Tachycardia is a heart rate of greater than 100 beats per minute. When the heart beats too quickly, there is a shortened relaxation phase. This causes two main problems: the ventricles are unable to fill completely, causing cardiac output to decrease; and the coronary arteries receive less blood, causing supply to the heart to decrease.

- Tachycardia is classified as stable or unstable.
- Heart rates greater than or equal to 150 beats per minute usually cause symptoms.
- Unstable tachycardia always requires prompt attention.
- Stable tachycardia can become unstable.

SYMPTOMS OF TACHYCARDIA

- Hypotension
- Sweating
- Pulmonary edema/congestion
- Jugular venous distension

- Chest pain/discomfort
- Shortness of breath
- Weakness/dizziness/lightheadedness
- Altered mental state

SYMPTOMATIC TACHYCARDIA WITH HEART RATE > 100 BPM

1. **If the individual is unstable, provide immediate synchronized cardioversion.**
   - Is the individual's tachycardia producing hemodynamic instability and serious symptoms?
   - Are the symptoms (i.e., pain and distress of acute myocardial infarction (AMI)) producing the tachycardia?

2. **Assess the individual's hemodynamic status by establishing IV, giving supplementary oxygen and monitoring the heart.**
   - Heart rate of 100 to 130 bpm is usually result of underlying process and often represents sinus tachycardia. In sinus tachycardia, the goal is to identify and treat the underlying systemic cause.
   - Heart rate greater than 150 bpm may be symptomatic; the higher the rate, the more likely the symptoms are due to the tachycardia.

3. **Asses the QRS Complex.**

> *If at any point you become uncertain or uncomfortable during the treatment of a stable patient, seek expert consultation. The treatment of stable patients can be potentially harmful.*

> *Adenosine may cause bronchospasm; therefore, adenosine should be given with caution to patients with asthma.*

REGULAR NARROW COMPLEX TACHYCARDIA (PROBABLE SVT)

- Attempt vagal maneuvers.
- Obtain 12-lead ECG; consider expert consultation.
- Adenosine 6 mg rapid IVP; if no conversion, give 12 mg IVP (second dose); may attempt 12 mg once.

>> Next: Tachycardia Continued

IRREGULAR NARROW COMPLEX TACHYCARDIA (PROBABLE A-FIB)

- Obtain 12-lead ECG; consider expert consultation.
- Control rate with diltiazem 15 to 20 mg (0.25 mg/kg) IV over two minutes or beta-blockers.

REGULAR WIDE COMPLEX TACHYCARDIA (PROBABLE VT)

- Obtain 12-lead ECG; consider expert consultation.
- Convert rhythm using amiodarone 150 mg IV over 10 minutes.
- Perform elective cardioversion.

IRREGULAR WIDE COMPLEX TACHYCARDIA

- Obtain 12-lead ECG; consider expert consultation.
- Consider anti-arrhythmic.
- If Torsades de Pointes, give magnesium sulfate 1 to 2 gm IV; may follow with 0.5 to 1 gm over 60 minutes.

STABLE AND UNSTABLE TACHYCARDIA

RULES FOR SINUS TACHYCARDIA

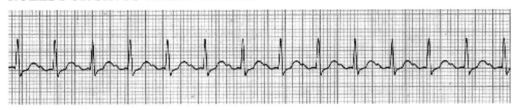

Figure 37

REGULARITY	*R-R intervals are regular, overall rhythm is regular.*
RATE	*The rate is over 100 bpm but usually less than 170 bpm.*
P WAVE	*There is one P wave in front of every QRS. The P waves appear uniform.*
PR INTERVAL	*Measures between 0.12-0.20 seconds in duration. PR interval is consistent.*
QRS COMPLEX	*Measures less than 0.12 seconds.*

Table 15

>> Next: Rules for Atrial Flutter

RULES FOR ATRIAL FLUTTER

RULES FOR ATRIAL FIBRILLATION (A-FIB) IRREGULAR NARROW COMPLEX TACHYCARDIA = A-FIB

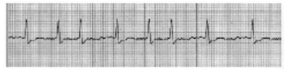

Figure 38

REGULARITY	*The atrial rate is regular. The ventricular rate will usually be regular, but only if the AV node conducts the impulses in a consistent manner. Otherwise, the ventricular rate will be irregular.*
RATE	*The atrial rate is normally between 250 to 350. Ventricular rate depends on conduction through the AV node to the ventricles.*
P WAVE	*The P waves will be well defined and have a "sawtooth" pattern to them.*
PR INTERVAL	*Due to the unusual configuration of P waves, the interval is not measured with atrial flutter.*
QRS COMPLEX	*QRS measures less than 0.12 seconds.*

Table 15 & 16

Figure 39

REGULARITY	*The R-R intervals are irregular; therefore, overall rhythm is irregularly irregular. The ventricles conduct from different atrial foci causing the irregularity.*
RATE	*Atrial rate usually exceeds 350. If the ventricular rate is between 60 and 100 bpm, this is known as "controlled" A-Fib. If the ventricular rate is more than 100, it is considered A-Fib with Rapid Ventricular Response (RVR), also known as uncontrolled A-Fib.*
P WAVE	*Due to the atria firing so rapidly from multiple foci, there are no obvious P waves in the rhythm. The baseline appears chaotic because the atria are fibrillating, therefore no P waves are produced.*
PR INTERVAL	*Because there are no P waves, PR interval cannot be measured.*
QRS COMPLEX	*QRS measures less than 0.12 seconds.*

>> Next: Adult Tachycardia with Pulse Algorithm

Adult Tachycardia with Pulse Algorithm

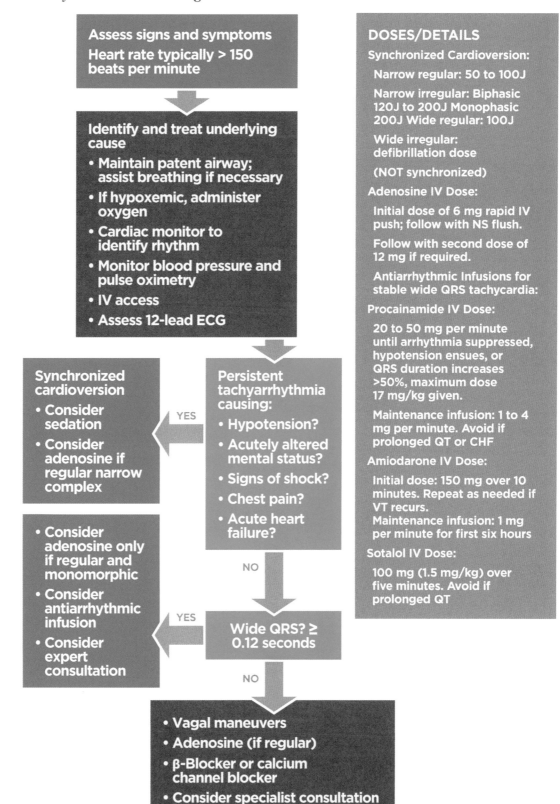

Figure 40

>> Next: Acute Coronary Syndrome

ACUTE CORONARY SYNDROME

Acute coronary syndrome (ACS) is a collection of clinical presentations including unstable angina, non-ST-elevation myocardial infarction (NSTEMI) and ST-elevation myocardial infarction (STEMI). ACS is classically recognized by one or more of the following symptoms: crushing chest pain, shortness of breath, pain that radiates to the jaw, arm or shoulder, sweating, and/or nausea or vomiting. It is important to note that not all individuals with ACS will present with these classic findings, particularly women and individuals with diabetes mellitus. It is impossible to determine a specific cardiac event from the ACS symptoms; therefore, ACS symptoms are managed in the same way.

Every individual with these symptoms should be evaluated immediately. If an individual appears to be unconscious, begin with the BLS Survey and follow the appropriate pathway for advanced care. If the individual is conscious, proceed with the pathway below.

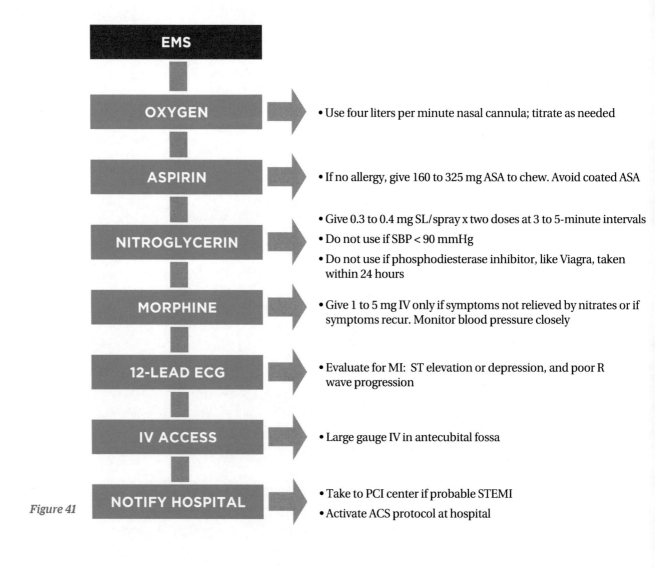

EMS

OXYGEN
• Use four liters per minute nasal cannula; titrate as needed

ASPIRIN
• If no allergy, give 160 to 325 mg ASA to chew. Avoid coated ASA

NITROGLYCERIN
• Give 0.3 to 0.4 mg SL/spray x two doses at 3 to 5-minute intervals
• Do not use if SBP < 90 mmHg
• Do not use if phosphodiesterase inhibitor, like Viagra, taken within 24 hours

MORPHINE
• Give 1 to 5 mg IV only if symptoms not relieved by nitrates or if symptoms recur. Monitor blood pressure closely

12-LEAD ECG
• Evaluate for MI: ST elevation or depression, and poor R wave progression

IV ACCESS
• Large gauge IV in antecubital fossa

NOTIFY HOSPITAL
• Take to PCI center if probable STEMI
• Activate ACS protocol at hospital

Figure 41

>> *Next: Acute Coronary Syndrome Algorithm*

Adult Coronary Syndrome Algorithm

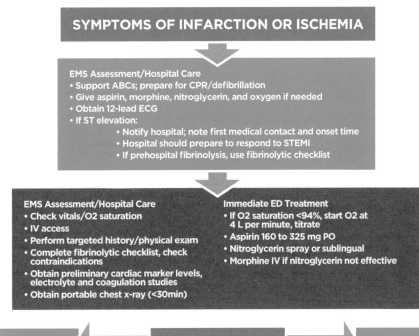

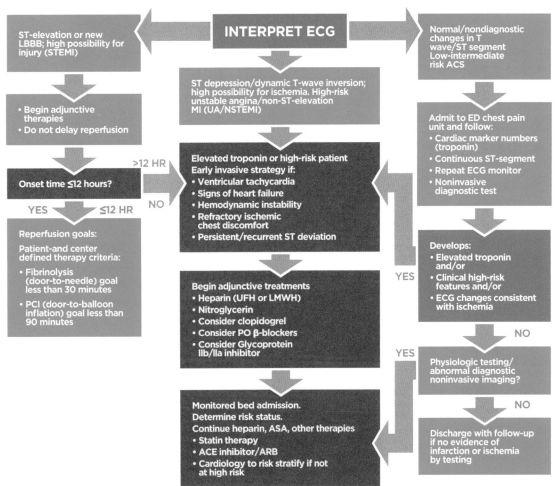

SYMPTOMS OF INFARCTION OR ISCHEMIA

EMS Assessment/Hospital Care
• Support ABCs; prepare for CPR/defibrillation
• Give aspirin, morphine, nitroglycerin, and oxygen if needed
• Obtain 12-lead ECG
• If ST elevation:
 • Notify hospital; note first medical contact and onset time
 • Hospital should prepare to respond to STEMI
 • If prehospital fibrinolysis, use fibrinolytic checklist

EMS Assessment/Hospital Care
• Check vitals/O2 saturation
• IV access
• Perform targeted history/physical exam
• Complete fibrinolytic checklist, check contraindications
• Obtain preliminary cardiac marker levels, electrolyte and coagulation studies
• Obtain portable chest x-ray (<30min)

Immediate ED Treatment
• If O2 saturation <94%, start O2 at 4 L per minute, titrate
• Aspirin 160 to 325 mg PO
• Nitroglycerin spray or sublingual
• Morphine IV if nitroglycerin not effective

ST-elevation or new LBBB; high possibility for injury (STEMI)

INTERPRET ECG

Normal/nondiagnostic changes in T wave/ST segment Low-intermediate risk ACS

• Begin adjunctive therapies
• Do not delay reperfusion

ST depression/dynamic T-wave inversion; high possibility for ischemia. High-risk unstable angina/non-ST-elevation MI (UA/NSTEMI)

Admit to ED chest pain unit and follow:
• Cardiac marker numbers (troponin)
• Continuous ST-segment
• Repeat ECG monitor
• Noninvasive diagnostic test

>12 HR

Elevated troponin or high-risk patient
Early invasive strategy if:
• Ventricular tachycardia
• Signs of heart failure
• Hemodynamic instability
• Refractory ischemic chest discomfort
• Persistent/recurrent ST deviation

Onset time ≤12 hours?

NO

YES ≤12 HR

Reperfusion goals:
Patient-and center defined therapy criteria:
• Fibrinolysis (door-to-needle) goal less than 30 minutes
• PCI (door-to-balloon inflation) goal less than 90 minutes

Develops:
• Elevated troponin and/or
• Clinical high-risk features and/or
• ECG changes consistent with ischemia

YES

Begin adjunctive treatments
• Heparin (UFH or LMWH)
• Nitroglycerin
• Consider clopidogrel
• Consider PO β-blockers
• Consider Glycoprotein IIb/IIa inhibitor

NO

YES

Physiologic testing/abnormal diagnostic noninvasive imaging?

Monitored bed admission.
Determine risk status.
Continue heparin, ASA, other therapies
• Statin therapy
• ACE inhibitor/ARB
• Cardiology to risk stratify if not at high risk

NO

Discharge with follow-up if no evidence of infarction or ischemia by testing

Figure 42

>> Next: Acute Stroke

ACUTE STROKE

Stroke is a condition in which normal blood flow to the brain is interrupted. Strokes can occur in two variations: ischemic and hemorrhagic. In ischemic stroke, a clot lodges in one of the brain's blood vessels, blocking blood flow through the blood vessel. In hemorrhagic stroke, a blood vessel in the brain ruptures, spilling blood into the brain tissue. Ischemic stroke and hemorrhagic stroke account for 87% and 13% of the total incidents, respectively. In general, the symptoms of ischemic and hemorrhagic strokes are similar. However, the treatments are very different.

SYMPTOMS OF STROKE

- Weakness in the arm and leg or face
- Vision problems
- Confusion
- Nausea or vomiting
- Trouble speaking or forming the correct words
- Problems walking or moving
- Severe headache (hemorrhagic)

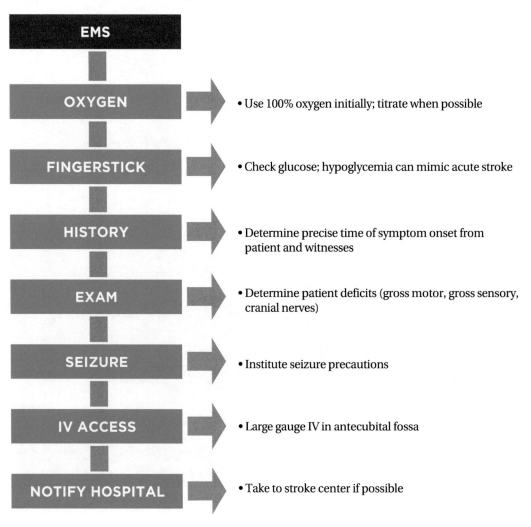

EMS

OXYGEN → • Use 100% oxygen initially; titrate when possible

FINGERSTICK → • Check glucose; hypoglycemia can mimic acute stroke

HISTORY → • Determine precise time of symptom onset from patient and witnesses

EXAM → • Determine patient deficits (gross motor, gross sensory, cranial nerves)

SEIZURE → • Institute seizure precautions

IV ACCESS → • Large gauge IV in antecubital fossa

NOTIFY HOSPITAL → • Take to stroke center if possible

Figure 43

>> Next: Acute Stroke Continued

Clinical signs of stroke depend on the region of the brain affected by decreased or blocked blood flow. Signs and symptoms can include: weakness or numbness of the face, arm, or leg, difficulty walking, difficulty with balance, vision loss, slurred or absent speech, facial droop, headache, vomiting, and change in level of consciousness. Not all of these symptoms are present, and the exam findings depend on the cerebral artery affected.

The Cincinnati Prehospital Stroke Scale (CPSS) is used to diagnose the presence of stroke in an individual if any of the following physical findings are seen: facial droop, arm drift, or abnormal speech. Individuals with one of these three findings as a new event have a 72% probability of an ischemic stroke. If all three findings are present, the probability of an acute stroke is more than 85%. Becoming familiar and proficient with the tool utilized by the rescuers' EMS system is recommended. Mock scenarios and practice will facilitate the use of these valuable screening tools.

Individuals with ischemic stroke who are not candidates for fibrinolytic therapy should receive aspirin unless contraindicated by true allergy to aspirin. All individuals with confirmed stroke should be admitted to Neurologic Intensive Care Unit if available. Stroke treatment includes blood pressure monitoring and regulation per protocol, seizure precautions, frequent neurological checks, airway support as needed, physical/occupational/speech therapy evaluation, body temperature, and blood glucose monitoring. Individuals who received fibrinolytic therapy should be followed for signs of bleeding or hemorrhage. Certain individuals (age 18 to 79 years with mild to moderate stroke) may be able to receive tPA (tissue plasminogen activator) up to 4.5 hours after symptom onset. Under certain circumstances, intra-arterial tPA is possible up to six hours after symptom onset. When the time of symptom onset is unknown, it is considered an automatic exclusion for tPA. If time of symptom onset is known, the National Institute of Neurological Disorders and Stroke (NINDS) has established the time goals below.

Figure 44

10 MINUTES OF ARRIVAL	**25 MINUTES OF ARRIVAL**	**60 MINUTES OF ARRIVAL**	**180 MINUTES OF ARRIVAL**
• General assessment by expert • Order urgent CT scan without contrast	• Perform CT scan without contrast • Neurological assessment • Read CT scan within 45 minutes	• Evaluate criteria for use and administer fibrinolytic therapy ("clot buster") • Fibrinolytic therapy may be used within three hours of symptom onset (4.5 hours in some cases)	• Admission to stroke unit

 Take Note

• Before giving anything (medication or food) by mouth, you must perform a bedside swallow screening. All acute stroke individuals are considered NPO on admission.

• The goal of the stroke team, emergency physician, or other experts should be to assess the individual with suspected stroke within 10 minutes of arrival in the emergency department (ED).

• The CT scan should be completed within 25 minutes of the individual's arrival in the ED and should be read within 45 minutes.

>> *Next: Emergency Department Staff*

EMERGENCY DEPARTMENT STAFF

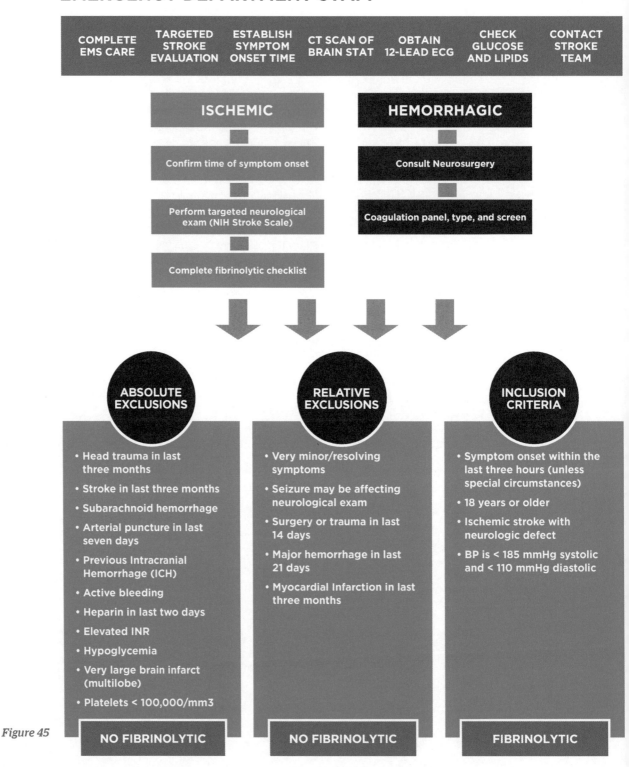

| COMPLETE EMS CARE | TARGETED STROKE EVALUATION | ESTABLISH SYMPTOM ONSET TIME | CT SCAN OF BRAIN STAT | OBTAIN 12-LEAD ECG | CHECK GLUCOSE AND LIPIDS | CONTACT STROKE TEAM |

ISCHEMIC

Confirm time of symptom onset

Perform targeted neurological exam (NIH Stroke Scale)

Complete fibrinolytic checklist

HEMORRHAGIC

Consult Neurosurgery

Coagulation panel, type, and screen

ABSOLUTE EXCLUSIONS

- Head trauma in last three months
- Stroke in last three months
- Subarachnoid hemorrhage
- Arterial puncture in last seven days
- Previous Intracranial Hemorrhage (ICH)
- Active bleeding
- Heparin in last two days
- Elevated INR
- Hypoglycemia
- Very large brain infarct (multilobe)
- Platelets < 100,000/mm3

NO FIBRINOLYTIC

RELATIVE EXCLUSIONS

- Very minor/resolving symptoms
- Seizure may be affecting neurological exam
- Surgery or trauma in last 14 days
- Major hemorrhage in last 21 days
- Myocardial Infarction in last three months

NO FIBRINOLYTIC

INCLUSION CRITERIA

- Symptom onset within the last three hours (unless special circumstances)
- 18 years or older
- Ischemic stroke with neurologic defect
- BP is < 185 mmHg systolic and < 110 mmHg diastolic

FIBRINOLYTIC

Figure 45

>> *Next: Acute Stroke Algorithm*

Acute Stroke Algorithm

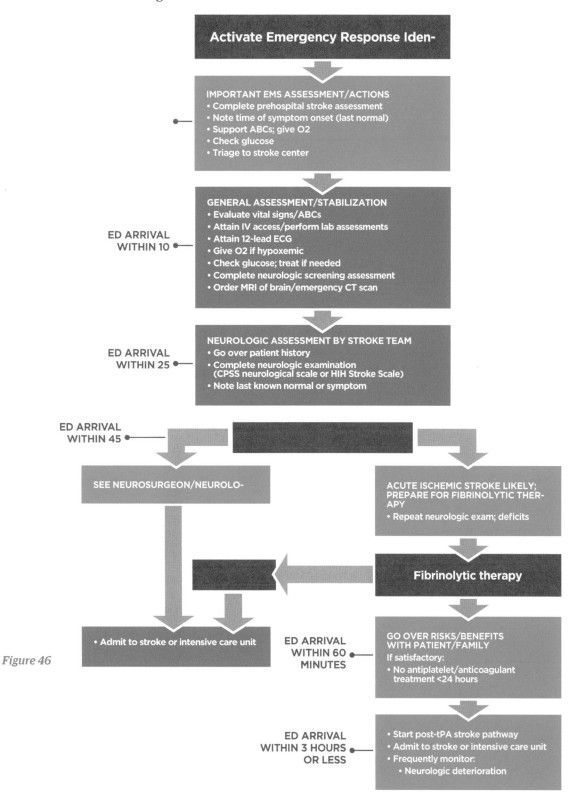

Figure 46

Activate Emergency Response Iden-

IMPORTANT EMS ASSESSMENT/ACTIONS
• Complete prehospital stroke assessment
• Note time of symptom onset (last normal)
• Support ABCs; give O2
• Check glucose
• Triage to stroke center

ED ARRIVAL WITHIN 10

GENERAL ASSESSMENT/STABILIZATION
• Evaluate vital signs/ABCs
• Attain IV access/perform lab assessments
• Attain 12-lead ECG
• Give O2 if hypoxemic
• Check glucose; treat if needed
• Complete neurologic screening assessment
• Order MRI of brain/emergency CT scan

ED ARRIVAL WITHIN 25

NEUROLOGIC ASSESSMENT BY STROKE TEAM
• Go over patient history
• Complete neurologic examination
  (CPSS neurological scale or HIH Stroke Scale)
• Note last known normal or symptom

ED ARRIVAL WITHIN 45

SEE NEUROSURGEON/NEUROLO-

ACUTE ISCHEMIC STROKE LIKELY; PREPARE FOR FIBRINOLYTIC THERAPY
• Repeat neurologic exam; deficits

Fibrinolytic therapy

• Admit to stroke or intensive care unit

ED ARRIVAL WITHIN 60 MINUTES

GO OVER RISKS/BENEFITS WITH PATIENT/FAMILY
If satisfactory:
• No antiplatelet/anticoagulant treatment <24 hours

ED ARRIVAL WITHIN 3 HOURS OR LESS

• Start post-tPA stroke pathway
• Admit to stroke or intensive care unit
• Frequently monitor:
  • Neurologic deterioration

SELF-ASSESSMENT FOR ACLS CASES

1. Which of the following is the correct next step in management after delivery of a shock?

    a. Check pulse.
    b. Ventilate only.
    c. Do chest compressions.
    d. Shock again.

2. Where does the electrical impulse for normal cardiac activity originate?

    a. Unknown
    b. SA node
    c. AV node
    d. Purkinje fibers

3. Choose the correct sequence of electrical activity in the heart for normal sinus rhythm?

    a. SA node, Purkinje, AV node, Bundle of His
    b. Purkinje, Bundle of His, AV node, SA node
    c. SA node, AV node, Bundle of His, Purkinje fibers
    d. AV node, SA node, Bundle of Hers, Purkinje fibers

4. What does the QRS complex on an ECG represent?

    a. Ventricular contraction
    b. AV valve closure
    c. Atrial contraction
    d. Septum relaxation

5. What is the recommended method to monitor breathing during ACLS care?

    a. Look, listen, and feel
    b. Capnography
    c. Venous blood gas
    d. Monitoring chest rise

6. You are transporting an individual who goes into cardiac arrest during transport. IV access is unsuccessful. What is the next step?

    a. Terminate resuscitation.
    b. Obtain intraosseous access.
    c. Place a central line.
    d. Administer all medications through ET tube.

7. Which vasopressin dose do you use to replace epinephrine during cardiac arrest?

    a. 10 mg
    b. 10 units
    c. 40 mg
    d. 40 units

8. An individual has been ill, and the monitor reveals sinus tachycardia with a heart rate of 135. What is the primary goal in treating this individual?

    a. Determine the underlying cause.
    b. Prepare for synchronized cardioversion.
    c. Transfuse packed red blood cells.
    d. Do adenosine administration.

9. A 79-year-old individual is in SVT. BP is 80/50, and he is complaining of chest discomfort and feels like passing out. What is the next appropriate step?

    a. Carotid massage
    b. Synchronized cardioversion
    c. Amiodarone
    d. Lidocaine

10. You are treating an individual who presented in ventricular fibrillation. After CPR and one attempt at defibrillation, his new rhythm is third-degree AV block. What is the next step in management?

    a. Repeat defibrillation
    b. Vasopressin
    c. Transcutaneous pacing
    d. High dose epinephrine

11. A 55-year-old male has stroke symptoms, and the CT scan shows multilobar infarction (more than one-third of the cerebral hemisphere). What therapy is contraindicated?

    a. Oxygen
    b. Monitoring glucose
    c. Thrombolytic therapy
    d. Blood pressure monitoring

12. What piece of data is critical to obtain in all stroke individuals?

    a. Date of birth
    b. Hemoglobin A1c
    c. Bilateral arm blood pressure
    d. Time last seen normal

13. True or False: The goal of stroke care is to complete the ED initial evaluation within 10 minutes, the neurologic evaluation within 25 minutes of arrival, and have the head CT read within 45 minutes of arrival.

ANSWERS

1. C
CPR is resumed for two minutes before any reassessment is performed. Begin with compressions followed by ventilation in a 30:2 ratio.

2. B
The SA node generates electrical impulse in normal cardiac activity. The impulse then travels to the rest of the conduction system and facilitates contraction of the atria and ventricles.

3. C
Normal cardiac electrical impulse travels in a consistent pattern producing normal sinus rhythm.

4. A
The QRS represents ventricular contraction. The T wave represents repolarization of the ventricles.

5. B
Quantitative waveform capnography is the recommended method to assess breathing/ventilation during ACLS. In addition, pulse oximetry should be assessed, and clinical assessment plays a role as well.

6. B
An intraosseous line can be placed rapidly and is the next best route for drug delivery. Absorption after ET tube delivery is unreliable.

7. D
A dose of vasopressin of 40 units may be used in place of the first or second dose of epinephrine. Epinephrine is given 3 to 5 minutes after the last dose of vasopressin, if a vasopressor is clinically required.

8. A
The primary objective of treating sinus tachycardia is to determine the underlying cause. Appropriate treatment decisions can then be made.

9. B
This individual is symptomatic of hypotension and chest pain. Adenosine could be considered if IV access is already in place, while preparation is made for cardioversion. Carotid massage may cause complications in elderly individuals.

10. C
Transcutaneous pacing is indicated for Mobitz Type II second degree AV block, third-degree AV block, and bradycardia with symptomatic ventricular escape rhythm.

11. C
Thrombolytic therapy is contraindicated in large strokes that involve more than one-third of a cerebral hemisphere.

12. D
Eligibility for thrombolytic therapy hinges on the time of onset of symptoms. Current guidelines support administering tPA for eligible individuals with symptom onset of three hours or fewer. Selected individuals may be eligible for up to 4.5 hours from onset.

13. True
Stroke is a neurologic emergency and rapid evaluation and treatment may improve outcomes. The mantra "Time is Brain" should be used here.

3 ACLS ESSENTIALS

- Prompt recognition and intervention with high-quality CPR is critical in any arrest situation.

- Mentally prepare for resuscitation as you approach the scene and the individual.

- Scene safety is critical; do not get injured yourself.

- BLS focus is early CPR and early defibrillation.

- Do not attempt to place an oropharyngeal airway in an awake individual.

- Pull the jaw up into the mask; do not push the mask onto the face as it may close the airway.

- IV or IO is the preferred routes for drug delivery; ET tube absorption is unpredictable.

- The dose of amiodarone is different for VF and VT with a pulse.

- Resume chest compressions immediately after delivering a shock.

- Therapeutic hypothermia is utilized after return of spontaneous circulation.

- Learn specific cardiac rhythms: sinus tachycardia, SVT, atrial fibrillation/flutter, VF, VT, Torsades de Pointes, and asystole.

- Confirm asystole in two separate leads.

- VF and pulseless VT are treated the same: deliver a shock.

- Remember the causes of PEA: the H's and the T's.

- Capnography is a valuable tool in resuscitation. If PETCO2 is greater than 10, attempt to improve CPR quality.

- Use nitroglycerin with caution in individuals with inferior myocardial infarction; avoid if systolic blood pressure (SBP) is less than 90 to 100, or if taking erectile dysfunction medications (phosphodiesterase inhibitors) within 24 hours.

- Confusion, nausea, and vomiting may be presenting signs of a stroke.

>> *Next: Additional Tools*

9 ADDITIONAL TOOLS

MEDICODE

With MediCode, you no longer will have to carry a set of expandable cards with you at all times while at work. You will never have to waste valuable time in an emergency situation searching through multiple algorithms until you find the right one. All of the algorithms are now accessible from the palm of your hand, and you will be selecting your desired algorithm by memory in no time. Choose between multiple viewing options and easily share algorithms with co-workers and friends through email and social media.

To improve functionality and speed in obtaining your desired algorithm as quickly as possible in an emergency, they have been divided between BLS, ACLS, PALS, and CPR. All are accessible from the home screen. The individual algorithms included in this app are:

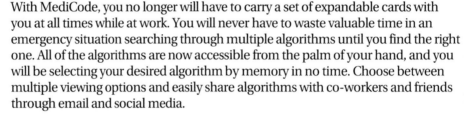

- Basic Life Support (BLS)
- Advanced Cardiac Life Support (ACLS)
- Pediatric Advanced Life Support (PALS)
- Cardiopulmonary Resuscitation (CPR) AED, and First Aid

CERTALERT+

CertAlert+ is the perfect app to minimize a potential area of stress and distraction in your life. With CertAlert+, you will have all your licenses and certifications in one place anytime you need them. We will keep track and remind you when your expiration date approaches, and we will help you with your registration whenever possible.

With CertAlert+, you can:

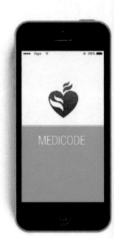

- Compile all required licenses and certifications in one location.
- Take photos (front and back) of certification cards and licenses for simple reference.
- Record all expiration dates and store with ease.
- Choose when you want to be reminded of your approaching expiration dates.
- Send all license or certification information directly to your email after exporting from the app.
- Quick access to easily register for online certification and recertification courses.

1. The following are included in the ACLS Survey:

    a. Airway, Breathing, Circulation, Differential Diagnosis
    b. Airway, Breathing, Circulation, Defibrillation
    c. Assessment, Breathing, Circulation, Defibrillation
    d. Airway, Breathing, CPR, Differential Diagnosis

2. The primary focus of cardiac arrest is:

    a. Effective CPR
    b. Early defibrillation
    c. Drug administration
    d. Both A and B

3. Which of the following is not an example of an advanced airway?

    a. Oropharyngeal airway
    b. Esophageal-tracheal tube
    c. Laryngeal mask airway
    d. Combitube

4. The following are possible effects of hyperventilation:

    a. Increased intrathoracic pressure
    b. Decreased venous return to the heart
    c. Both A and B
    d. None of the above

5. The normal sinus rhythm of the heart starts in the:

    a. Left ventricle
    b. Atrioventricular node
    c. Sinoatrial node
    d. Right ventricle

6. What is high-quality CPR?

    a. 80 compressions per minute at a depth of at least one-inch
    b. 100 to 120 compressions per minute at a depth of at 2 to 2.4 inches (5 to 6 cm)
    c. 80 compressions per minute at a depth of at least two inches
    d. 100 compressions per minute at a depth of at least one inch

7. Before placement of an advanced airway, the compression to ventilation ratio during CPR is:

    a. 30:1
    b. 30:2
    c. 15:1
    d. 20:2

8. You should_____ in an individual with ventricular fibrillation immediately following a shock.

    a. Resume CPR
    b. Check heart rate
    c. Analyze rhythm
    d. Give amiodarone

9. _____ joules (J) are delivered per shock when using a monophasic defibrillator.

    a. 200
    b. 260
    c. 300
    d. 360

10. The following medication(s) can be used to treat hypotension during the post-cardiac arrest phase:

    a. Dopamine
    b. Milrinone
    c. Amiodarone
    d. Both A and B

11. The following antiarrhythmic drug(s) can be used for persistent ventricular fibrillation or pulseless ventricular tachycardia, except:

    a. Amiodarone
    b. Lidocaine
    c. Atropine
    d. Both A and B

12. Which of the following is not a potential cause of PEA?

    a. Toxins
    b. Hyperkalemia
    c. Hyperventilation
    d. Trauma

13. Which of the following is a shockable rhythm?

    a. Ventricular fibrillation
    b. Ventricular tachycardia (pulseless)
    c. Torsades de Pointes
    d. All of the above

14. Which ACLS drug(s) may not be given via endotracheal tube?

    a. Naloxone
    b. Atropine
    c. Vasopressin
    d. Amiodarone

15. The following drug(s) may be used in an ACS individual for cardiac reperfusion:

    a. Fibrinolytic therapy
    b. Epinephrine
    c. Atropine
    d. Both A and C

16. All of the following are bradycardic rhythms except:

    a. Atrial fibrillation
    b. First-degree heart block
    c. Mobitz Type I
    d. Third-degree heart block

17. _____ access is preferred in arrest due to easy access and no interruption in CPR.

    a. Central
    b. Peripheral
    c. Intraosseous
    d. Endotracheal

18. Which of the following is first-line treatment for ACS?

    a. Morphine
    b. Aspirin
    c. Nitroglycerin
    d. All of the above

19. The following are classic signs of an acute stroke except:

    a. Facial droop
    b. Arm drift
    c. Abnormal speech
    d. All of the above

20. Which of the following is not found within the 8 D's of stroke care?

    a. Detection
    b. Dispatch
    c. Delivery
    d. Defibrillate

ANSWERS

1. A
   Airway, Breathing, Circulation, Differential Diagnosis

2. D
   Both A and B

3. A
   Oropharyngeal airway

4. C
   Both A and B

5. C
   Sinoatrial node

6. B
   100 to 120 compressions per minute at a depth of 2 to 2.4 inches (5 to 6 cm)

7. B
   30:2

ANSWERS continued

8. A
   Resume CPR

9. D
   360

10. A
    Dopamine

11. C
    Atropine

12. C
    Hyperventilation

13. D
    All of the above

14. D
    Amiodarone

15. A
    Fibrinolytic therapy

16. A
    Atrial fibrillation

17. B
    Peripheral

18. D
    All of the above

19. D.
    All of the above

20. D
    Defibrillate

Made in the USA
Coppell, TX
21 April 2020

21230768R00045